gorge

MY JOURNEY UP KILIMANJARO AT 300 POUNDS

Kara Richardson Whitely

SEAL PRESS

THANK YOU FOR JOINING ME on this journey.

This is a memoir, my truth of my life as a plus-size adventurer. I used documentary footage, journals, interviews, and memory to retrace my steps through childhood and up Africa's highest peak. Some names have been changed to protect privacy. Some have not.

Filmmakers Sharon Dennis of Reel World Productions and Sydney Clover, who was a film student at the time, joined us on this journey up Mount Kilimanjaro to document it. In true journalistic fashion, other than a few microphone adjustments and such, they did not interject or interfere in the story.

So please, come along with me. We have amazing places to go.

HAPPY TRAILS,
KARA

GORGE
Copyright © 2015 Kara Richardson Whitely

SEAL PRESS
A Member of the Perseus Books Group
1700 Fourth Street
Berkeley, California 94710

Library of Congress Cataloging-in-Publication Data

Whitely, Kara Richardson.
  Gorge : my journey up Kilimanjaro at 300 pounds / by Kara Richardson Whitely.
      pages cm
  "Distributed by Publishers Group West"—T.p. verso.
  ISBN 978-1-58005-559-8
1. Whitely, Kara Richardson. 2. Women mountaineers—United States—Biography. 3. Mountaineering—Tanzania—Kilimanjaro, Mount. I. Title.
  GV199.92.W463A3 2015
  796.52092—dc23
  [B]
                              2014036176

10 9 8 7 6 5 4 3 2 1

Cover design by Erin Seaward-Hiatt
Cover photo © Sally Kidd. After four days of hiking, author Kara Richardson Whitely and hiking partner Stacey make the final approach for summit night on Africa's highest peak, Mt. Kilimanjaro.
Interior design by Domini Dragoone

Printed in the United States of America
Distributed by Publishers Group West

For Chris, Anna, and Emily, you are the stars in my sky

Table of Contents

It is not the mountain we conquer, but ourselves.
—*Sir Edmund Hillary, first man to summit Mount Everest*

Prologue

TANZANIA, AFRICA

I WAS THE FATTEST HIKER on the mountain, and I was in trouble.

It was 3:00 AM on the morning of our Mount Kilimanjaro summit attempt, and our group of four women—all friends, all of us raising money for Global Alliance for Africa's AIDS orphans programs—had dwindled to three. I wondered if I would be next.

We were so high up that the stars were not only above but also beside and below us. To be among the stars was a wondrous feeling after so many years weighed down by my fears, too scared to put myself out into the world, to be seen.

The headlamps of other hikers looked like constellations moving in formation as they passed us on the gravelly, zigzag trail. We had started at 11:00 PM, an hour earlier than most groups, to get a jump on the summit attempt. But we were already behind on this day of fifteen hours of hiking more than 19,000 feet up Africa's highest peak.

With each step, I felt as if I was dying. My lungs seethed and prayed for air. My legs were lead. My heart beat so hard and fast against my ribcage that I thought it might leap out onto the frozen ground below.

Our group took breaks every half hour—more than most others—and I worried that I was the one holding everyone back. We found a spot to pause at Williams Point—an outcropping of rocks at 16,400 feet where summit-seekers can rest for no longer than a few minutes. Otherwise, at ten degrees, fingers and other body parts could freeze. I was too exhausted to be hungry, but in hopes of restoring some of my energy, I reached into the outside pocket of my backpack for a Clif Bar and discovered that it was frozen. I gnawed and gnawed but couldn't even break off a nibble.

I had always relied on food to get me through adversity. Now, when I really needed to eat, I couldn't.

My headlamp illuminated my breath, each exhalation like a frosty jellyfish in the dark, suspended for a moment, and then slipping into darkness. I was scared to let my breath escape, wondering if the next would provide me with enough oxygen to keep me going. Near Kilimanjaro's summit, there is half as much oxygen as at sea level. Standing still at Williams Point, with another 2,000 feet to go, I was panting like a chubby middle school student who had just finished the mile run.

You might wonder what a fat person was doing climbing Mount Kilimanjaro. And when I say I'm fat, I'm not being charmingly self-deprecating. Each of my legs was the width of a century-old tree. My hips were as wide as a Smart car bumper. I had to sit on buckets instead of camping chairs for fear that the fabric would rip and I would land on the ground, humiliated.

I weighed three hundred pounds. I was a glutton, plain and simple, as well as a glutton for punishment. This was my third trek up the mountain.

CHAPTER 1

Uphill Battle

SECOND SUMMIT ATTEMPT, TWO YEARS EARLIER, DECEMBER 2009: MARANGU, TANZANIA, 6,496 FEET

My hair was damp the second I stuck my head out of my window at the Kilimanjaro Mountain Resort. I wanted to have a glimpse of the 19,343-foot mountain before me, but it remained elusive, hidden behind the gray drifting mist that consumed the sky and soaked the red volcanic earth below.

The tour book said the rainy season ended in early December, but here in the week before Christmas, Mother Nature did not seem to agree.

I didn't need to see Mount Kilimanjaro after all. I already knew it looked a lot like my own generous pear figure: boxy and wide at the bottom. I had already trodden to its summit once two years prior to celebrate a 120-pound weight loss.

I thought retracing those steps would be enough to get me back on track. I desperately wanted to return to the one time I felt I had my weight under control. The first path to Kilimanjaro started after tackling Camel's Hump in Vermont, a peak that had defeated me during college, on my thirty-first birthday. I had just crossed over the 300-pound mark. I spent a year resisting carbs and starting each day with a two-hour workout. Taking on Mount Kilimanjaro, the highest nontechnical mountain one could reach the top of by hiking, was a reward for finally dipping below 300 pounds to a low of 240 (size twenty-four).

I was feeling my strongest and most in control. People who knew me at my fattest called me "skinny." Men held doors for me. I felt as radiant as the first sunrise over Kilimanjaro's sister peak, Mawenzi, which illuminated all of Africa below. I could buy shirts and jackets at the Gap, something I could have never done in my plus-size life.

That first time, I bounded to Kilimanjaro's Uhuru Peak at 19,343 feet with energy to spare. This second time, I was once again standing at the base of Mount Kilimanjaro, but I wasn't in the same place. This time, having given birth to a daughter, Anna, I didn't do the training. I didn't drop the pounds. I didn't deserve to be here. I told myself not to panic. I'm really great at high altitude. It was just a very long walk to the top of the mountain.

After gaining more than half of my weight back after the first Kilimanjaro climb, I was there for the second time in hopes of dropping pounds, but I really should have done that before arriving in Marangu, the village at the base of the mountain. This time, instead of taking a hike as a celebration, the trek felt more like a condemnation.

I looked back at my duffle bag, which was just as stuffed as my size twenty-eight jeans. I had packed the same things as last time, ignoring the fact I had gained seventy pounds while pregnant and in the months after life with my daughter.

I hesitated in terror.

Wait, did I even try on my pants? I remembered sticking both pairs in the bag, trying to ignore that size 3X might not fit me anymore. The last time I wore them, they were roomy, and I needed to use the canvas belt woven through the waistband to keep them up.

A moment of panic set over me as I unzipped my duffle bag, its contents nearly spilling out of the overstuffed sack. My heart pounded. I may be about to set off on a seven-day journey on a mountain without proper pants.

I was sure I'd lose fifteen pounds while hiking, but that didn't matter before everything started. The two pant legs swished together as I held them up as if in prayer.

Please let these fit. Please let these fit.

I unzipped my jeans, letting them fall to the floor and straight into the rain puddle below the open window.

Stepping out of my soaked britches, I hung them on the wooden bedpost, hoping they would dry. "Shit, shit, shit," I said, trying to fan them, delaying my encounter with the hiking pants.

I sat down on the bed, trying on the slate-gray pair first. I looped my ankles in them the same way my ninety-year-old grandmother would get dressed.

Over the ankles. Check.

Over the knees. Check.

But as I stood to pull them up over my thighs, the waist wasn't a big enough circumference to pass. They stayed, pinching my bumpy cellulite. Each fiber of the fabric seemed to yelp as I tried to nudge them upward. A little on the right, a little on the left. But there was no way these pants would pass over my hips, which extended three feet wide. Wicking material, which is imperative on a mountain hike to stay dry and comfortable, isn't known for its stretch or give.

I pulled them down again, feverishly trying to unbuckle the canvas drawstring belt that came standard, completely unhooking it. But the results were the same. They were stuck on my thighs.

I sunk back down on the bed, the mattress sinking below me. I buried my head in my hands. Oh no. I'm so fucked.

My mind worked up every possible scenario to get around this, from feigning illness and flying right back to my husband and daughter to hiking the whole trek in jeans—which would be a disaster when the cotton-blend material would get soaked and stay that way to the top of the mountain.

I imagined myself trying to maneuver over the jagged Jamaica Rocks, the treacherous last challenge before arriving at the peak, in jeans frozen straight and solid.

I ripped the slate-gray pants off and I held them up to the sky by the waistband. I just need these to be bigger. I just needed to be smaller.

It was hard enough finding a pair of polyester pants in size thirty back home. While Marangu catered to people about to set foot on the mountain, there would be no plus-size hiking supplies. I was the fattest hiker most people had ever seen.

I remembered passing a hut with a sewing machine out front on the bumpy van ride to the hotel. I thought that must be a tailor.

I looked at the two pairs of pants. Since they were the same cut, I thought they could become one. It would just be a matter of adding six inches of fabric from one to the other. The problem was, they were different colors, one slate gray and the other sandy beige. The six-inch stripe of sandy beige extending from my hip to my ankle would be my scarlet letter. My shame for being too fat, as if my wide hips and bulging belly weren't enough.

I pulled on my sopping-wet jeans, looking like I peed my pants, and rushed down to the front desk. Arriving out of breath—not a great sign for the journey ahead—I asked the woman working there for a favor.

Laughing nervously, I told her, "I packed the wrong pants! Is there a tailor around who can cut six inches from these to add to the other?" I showed her my plan.

She nodded along and asked, "What should I do with the remaining smaller pants?"

"Oh, the tailor can keep those. They won't fit me," I said, immediately regretting that I said that aloud.

I handed her the equivalent of five dollars to do the job, mad that I had to spend what little money I had on fixing my fatness. I hoped it worked. If it didn't I would have nothing.

I returned to my room filled with worry that this wouldn't work and heavy with shame, embarrassment, and fear. I had signed up to hike the mountain to raise money for Global Alliance for Africa's AIDS orphans programs for the second time. I had dozens of sponsors and thousands of dollars in donations riding on this, and I'd already let them down. I'd let myself down. I'd let the children of Africa down. And I was only at the base of the mountain.

As these thoughts ate away at my ambition, my mind zeroed in on a purchase that I had made in Amsterdam, packed neatly in my suitcase.

When you climb Kilimanjaro, you pack two pieces of luggage. One duffle bag for the mountain. One suitcase for clean clothes before and after the trek.

In the layover at the Amsterdam airport, I'd purchased a gallon bag of miniature chocolates, Milky Way bars and the like. I thought they'd make lovely stocking stuffers for my daughter, niece, and nephew once I was home.

That's what I told myself again and again as I held them in the checkout line. I thought about putting them back, but I didn't. I couldn't release my grasp even as I paced back and forth in the store hoping I'd make a better decision.

I mentioned to the cashier, in an offhand way, "These are for my niece and nephew visiting from California."

She just nodded with a Dutch-accented "Sure, lady," kind of look.

I stuffed them in my carry-on suitcase, where they stayed all the way to Kilimanjaro International Airport.

The holiday candy plan unraveled that night in my hotel room. I was mortified, ashamed, afraid, and alone in my hotel room—except for the bag of candy.

I had eaten a healthy dinner of stew and felt full, yet I couldn't stop thinking of those miniature chocolates. Well, I could have just one, I thought. Then I'd leave the rest in my luggage. I'd zip it tight, maybe even secure it with the little luggage lock.

Hah. I've never had just one of anything in my life.

I opened the bag and plucked out a candy bar. Then one more. Then three more. Then I was lost in a haze of chocolate nougat and caramel. Like a pit bull tearing apart a steak, I just couldn't stop the frenzy.

In that moment between me and the candy bars, I was lost. Somewhere else. I was transported above and beyond the shaky start to the challenge of my second climb. My eating was mechanical, hand to mouth. Repeat. Repeat. Repeat. There was no stopping between the first bite and the last. I told myself, "I'll just have one more." It wasn't that I intended to overindulge. It just happened, an act beyond my body.

When it was over, I was restored to myself and plummeted into the bowels of shame. I had finished the bag, the entire gallon bag. All the shiny wrappers were winking at me from the garbage. Each and every one of those sweet little candy bars was gone. I had literally taken candy from children. Candy that was intended for children I love. I was a criminal.

So many of my binges started with the intention of doing something nice for someone else. That's what I wanted to believe anyway.

This is my husband's favorite ice cream.

My daughter will love this treat.

So few of the treats ever make it to the intended person.

The incredible thing is, I rarely enjoy the sweets I pilfer. They are a means to an end, a way to temporarily feed the beast of my food addiction, compulsive overeating, or whatever you want to call it. The only time I love, or even taste, food is when I eat it in the company of someone else. When I have to control myself.

That night, I was alone facing my own demons in a hotel room. I worried that one day I'd be found lying on the ground having choked to death on a butterscotch disk, like so many rock stars found dead of an overdose in a bathtub. But not this time.

There was a sick feeling in my stomach as it valiantly tried to process the sugar overload, as it had done so many times before. If my stomach could speak, it would be begging, "Please. That's enough."

Shifting into self-preservation, I wasn't thinking about my stomach anymore. I had to cover my tracks—or my bites. No one could know about this. I stuffed some tissues over the candy wrappers in the garbage. But I knew from the looks of all three hundred pounds of me, the woman in need of one pair of pants made from two, there was no hiding my deed. Besides, I was one of only three guests staying there. The staff would surely trace the wrappers to me. Everyone would know. I was just postponing the discovery of the evidence. The binge helped me escape reality for a moment, but the truth was still there.

I was about to hike forty miles. My already bloated stomach protruded more than usual, and I knew I wouldn't get a minute's sleep after all that chocolate—too much caffeine. Not a great way to begin my quest to Kilimanjaro's summit.

THE NEXT MORNING, THE RAIN clouds lifted, and I came down to the lobby to see the front desk woman in her perfectly tailored navy suit.

"Ah, we have your pants," she said, holding them out wide.

I wanted her to put them down at once. So others wouldn't see the britches that spread like a tent tarp in her outstretched arms.

"Thanks so much for handling that," I said, folding them quickly and tucking the layers of fabric under my arm. I went back to my room to try them on in privacy.

They fit. Thank God they fit. Or at least that's how I thought I was supposed to feel. Part of me wished they wouldn't fit so I'd have an excuse to go home and abandon all of this.

I sat through a breakfast of porridge and fruit, burping up the taste of chocolate. I wavered between feeling grateful that my pants fit and terrified it meant I'd actually have to go up the mountain.

I left the resort wearing the pants, feeling the new seam dig into my hips with every twist and turn in the road on the van ride to the trailhead. Our driver had to work to avoid children with shaved heads wearing royal blue or green school uniforms, who stopped mid-track to wave whenever they saw a tourist bus pass.

The first day on the trail, it rained so hard that the water soaked through our mess tent. I was soaked, sluggish, and miserable.

The second day on the trail, I threw up. I could taste chocolate.

After three more miserable, sluggish days, it all came to an end.

On the night we attempted the summit, my legs weren't doing what my brain was telling them to. I had promised my family that I would return home safe and sound. With less than three miles to the top, I turned back. Defeated.

Even though the thousands of dollars I raised would still go to charity, I was still fat. That fact made the whole trip feel like a failure. It made me feel like a failure.

Maybe I dropped ten pounds on the mountain, but I would find them again in airport kiosks and by finishing every last crumb of plane food.

Back home, I told my friends and family that I had picked up some kind of stomach bug, but I knew the real reason I had failed was that I was unprepared. I'd taken my body for granted. I had gone from being at the top of Kilimanjaro to the low point between two mountains—the gorge.

CHAPTER 2

Deep Woods

GANANOQUE, ONTARIO, CANADA, 1979

SOME KILIMANJARO BOOKS CALL THE trek a mere "walk to the summit." In certain circles, it's known as a tourist hike, an add-on to a safari. In truth, it is anything but.

Martha Stewart made it to the top of the mountain. Ann Curry did not. Martina Navratilova did not. Would I?

Foreigners have been trying to conquer Kilimanjaro since 1861 when German officer Carl Claus Von der Decken and British geologist Richard Thornton tried to ascend but got no more than 8,200 feet—not even halfway up the mountain. Relentless in his pursuit, Von der Decken tried again the following year with Otto Kersten, and reached about 14,000 feet, the height of many peaks in the Rockies, but only three-quarters of the way to Kilimanjaro's summit. With each attempt, the explorers learned something about the mountain and, I imagined, about themselves.

It may seem freakish that someone like me would take on the challenge, but given my rural upbringing and my love of nature, it wasn't actually that far-fetched.

I am lighthearted and heavy-footed. I'm half Swede from my mother, a quarter German and a quarter Irish from my father—and all Viking, prone to going on expeditions. This also means I am six feet tall, sturdy, and fair. Well, fair is putting it lightly. I essentially spontaneously combust after a few moments in the sun.

When I was younger, I found solace and shade with my two older brothers, Bryan and Derek, in the forest that was our front yard in Gananoque, a hamlet within the Thousand Islands region of Ontario. Bryan, who is four years older than I, used to fetch salamanders from the stream and let them loose in the house. Derek and I, just two years apart, would find them dried up behind the couch, as if they had been waiting to pounce on our shoulders.

The first signs of spring were the budding wildflowers, the trilliums and jack-in-the-pulpits, shoving through the thawing forest floor. The flowers were spots of white, purple, and yellow among the pungent ground, which smelled of pine needles and moist bark. As kids, we were left outside to be wild and free. I twirled in my gingham dress like Julie Andrews in *The Sound of Music*, arms stretched wide, until I was dizzy. I'd lie down and watch the sky circle around me.

In winters, we had a wood shed nearly two stories tall, jam-packed with logs and close enough to the house that we could get to it even in the worst of blizzards, which left snow walls taller than my four-year-old blond head. Inside, I watched the flicker of the fireplace and burrowed my head into my father's nubby blue robe, which smelled of many fires before, as we watched the dancing flames together.

My dad most often wore a white T-shirt, covering a jagged scar that stretched the length of his belly. It was from his time in Vietnam, where he had been shot and stabbed. I imagined the medics hurriedly stitching him up, with bullets flying overhead. There were other scars too, raised pink lines where he was cut open from surgeries he'd had since his return from war, including procedures after a massive heart attack he suffered on his own wedding day. He was given six months to live ten years previously. I'd look up from time to time and notice his gray-blue eyes were the same as mine.

I suppose we were survivalists, living in a summer cottage that became our full-time home. We communicated only by CB radio to the outside world.

To get to the bus stop in the winter, we had to travel by snowmobile. The snowmobile exhaust puffed out as my father pull-started it when I exited the house, with the front steps cleared just wide enough for us to leave. The rumble of the engine starting excited me as I hopped on behind him, my brothers piled on behind me.

I clutched the waist of Dad's parka tight with my mitten-covered hands and leaned my face against his back as the snowmobile zoomed through the silence of the mile-long hill, trees bending from the ice and snow. The scarf that my mother wrapped around my hood flopped in the tailwind of our journey to the school bus stop.

Back then, food was nothing more than nourishment to me.

My mother made jam from our own berries. I helped her stir the vat of deep red preserves, a simple mix of fruit, sugar, and pectin. She baked bread, too. I watched her pasty arms knead the dough. I sat in the kitchen to get a whiff of it slowly rising in a bowl covered with a kitchen cloth.

I'd come home to the smell of onions, carrots, and celery simmering in butter, the start of my mother's potato chowder. It was a Swedish family recipe with a pinch of tarragon.

My father had a thing for hi-fi systems so our place was wired for optimum sound, and an entire wall of the living room was lined with various albums. Dad liked jazz. My mother loved Abba, The Carpenters, Anne Murray, and John Denver.

During dinner, I watched the evening sun create rainbows on the ceiling as it passed by our stained-glass window and set over the South Lake, where we'd swim in the summer with pikes nipping at our toes like worms and my father shooed a menacing snapping turtle out of my mother's garden with a shovel.

The best time of the year was Christmas. My father loved celebrating, although he could hardly wait until the big day to share our gifts. One year, I got a candy cane almost as long as my arm, a wooden play hutch, and a pair of cross-country skis. When I tried on the skis to race down the slope next to our house, I took a big tumble. My legs ended up in a tangle. My mother came to the rescue.

"Oh, honey," she said, looking at my twisted body. She unraveled me, kissed my tears away, and helped me back up the hill to the kitchen, heated by a cast-iron woodstove. The smell of the fire was soothing and warm as I defrosted.

But one day, when I was eight years old, everything changed. We moved to upstate New York, to an eighty-two-acre property in a town outside Potsdam, for my father's continued studies in metallurgical engineering. Things felt hopeful at first. We had a phone and a television. My brothers, Bryan and Derek, loved the new place and particularly enjoyed walking to an abandoned sugar shack in the woods. I picked wildflowers as I went with them, tinkering with the rusted tin buckets and imagining what life would be like making my own syrup. Maybe someday I could get this sugar shack running again, even though there were holes in the wooden walls.

Our house wasn't much of a home, just something you might pass on a road trip without notice. The façade was burnt orange, the yard lined with sumacs. The linoleum floors were cold. My mom didn't do much to make things better. She hung a few of her favorite bird carvings and watercolor paintings, but left most of the walls bare.

What I didn't know then was my parents were on the verge of separation. I could tell something wasn't right with them; there were bouts of shouting followed by extended silences. I started noticing Dad wasn't home much. He was clearly having an affair, which of course I didn't know then. I thought he was just away for conferences and teaching. Once, my mother called me into her bedroom weeping, and had me get on the phone to beg my father to come home.

"Please come home, Daddy," I whimpered into the phone. I could smell his Old Spice on his pillow next to me on the bed. "Where are you?"

"Put your mother back on the phone," he snapped in a gruff voice that was only used to punish me.

I handed my mother the phone, her eyes reddened from crying for hours. Her demeanor was as if she'd been punched in the gut. She seemed exhausted from fighting the knowledge that my father was gone.

"Don't hang up on me," she screamed at the receiver, which now played the dial tone. She lay in fetal position in her bed, her legs clinging to the sheets as she wailed.

I lay with her, my head resting on her hip as she sobbed.

It was only later that I realized my dad had been with another woman named Helen, who would eventually become my stepmother. For the time being, things seemed to get better. My father came home. My parents seemed to do less shouting. But then, my father started to go away for long periods again. One Christmas, after rushing through dinner, he shined his shoes and went off to spend the rest of the holiday with Helen. The house and I felt empty.

WHEN MY FATHER'S FATHER LEFT him, his mother, and his sister, my dad was three years old. It would be a decade before my father saw him again; he was dying of lung cancer around that time. The invitation was to his deathbed, to say goodbye. But since it was the first time my father had seen him in a decade, he had nothing to say.

"That was my father," my dad said anytime he shared the story with us. He looked at me as if I should be grateful for all he was.

Even when he was a child, no place felt like home to my father. Every six months or so, he and his mother relocated, and it was his job to help fix the new houses up, hammering, sanding, and painting instead of playing. His mother married five times to try to stay afloat.

He once told me that each time he moved to a new school district, he made a point of finding the biggest, toughest kid and punching him in the face so he would be left alone for the duration of his short stay. By the time he was seventeen, he enlisted in the Army. He reenlisted in the Navy and stayed there long enough for Vietnam. Like many veterans, he wouldn't return as the same person. The only thing I know about his tour was that his friend was blown up right next to him.

"You just wouldn't want to know," he said once when I asked him if he wanted to talk about it. We knew not to awaken him by startling him or to sneak up behind him. In restaurants, he would only pick seats where his back wasn't facing the door.

"I'm a trained killer," he told us. While he never struck us, I never tested him on this.

So it probably doesn't come as a surprise that there was no "your mom and dad are getting a divorce" talk. My notice was my mother's

Ford Escort packed so tightly that it sagged low to the ground. Standing near the unstained railing of our porch, which wobbled with each step, I still didn't get it. I clung to my father, who wore his Navy SEALs T-shirt, begging my mom to leave me behind.

"What if I just stayed?" I cried, digging my fingernails into my father's sleeve.

"It's time to go," my mother said. "We're moving to Vermont."

"I don't even know where that is," I screeched into the wind. My hands flailed in the air. They didn't teach U.S. geography in Canada. I was nine years old but I sounded more like a toddler in the midst of a temper tantrum, fingernails now deepening into the wet wood of the porch. "I'm staying."

"It's just a few hours away," she said.

I could see my mother's reluctance to come near me while I was attached to my father. It was as if his aura was too hot, too painful to be near. But eventually, after I had grown hoarse from shouting, she came, took my hand, put her arm around my shoulder, and tugged me to the car.

I kicked the back of the driver's seat until my feet ached. My brother Derek, with his bowl-cut hair and glasses, just looked down at the floor of the car. Bryan, with his arm outside of the front passenger window, waved goodbye. I sobbed until the state line, and pressed my face against the frosted car window as we crossed over Lake Champlain.

CHAPTER 3

Hiker Girl

SUMMIT, NJ, 2010, ABOUT A YEAR BEFORE THE THIRD CLIMB CAME TO BE

It was a crisp, fall morning. The kind that begged for apple cider donuts. A hayride. Leaf peeping. Our bedroom was just cold enough to require an extra blanket.

As I rolled over in my king-size bed, I saw my daughter's hair, as blond as mine was as a kid. It fell softly on the pillow next to me. I let her drift off to sleep there at about three o'clock in the morning. She came in after another nightmare, which I had read was normal for three-year-olds. I let her nestle in, hoping this way I'd get some sleep. But I wasn't able to fall asleep again so I lay awake until 7:00 AM.

I remembered seeing an episode of *Caillou*, a Canadian children's show, where the perfect mom guided her son back to his room after a nightmare and turned over the pillow to the "good dream side," but that never seemed to work for me. I just wanted to go back to sleep. So our bed was often home to three: my husband Chris, my daughter, and me.

Her leg flopped over me as she rolled into my space, a concave etch of my rump. I rolled to my side, but she dug her head into my back trying to nuzzle more.

Between my daughter and my husband's diagonal pose, I was pushed to the last foot of the bed and decided it was time to get up.

My toes winced at the touch of the cold floor. I looped my size thirty black pants around my feet, which I bought as maternity wear four years prior, and stood, pulling them up with me. I figured those pants plus my ratty T-shirt were decent enough to wear to start the coffee. I didn't like to walk around without pants, exposing the blue varicose veins against my pasty skin, even if no one was around. The bumpy cellulite-ridden landscape of my thighs was unwelcoming. My granny-plus briefs covered as much as they could.

As I rose, the floor creaking below my feet, my husband awoke. He seemed to sniff the air and embrace the chill of sweatshirt-and-jeans weather that was so appealing to us. I grew up in Vermont. He attended Middlebury College. Simply put, we loved fall and everything about it.

"I could go for a pumpkin donut," Chris said with a yawn, plopping his feet on the ground and reaching for his glasses, folded next to a pile of books as high as the lampshade on his nightstand, to help his green eyes see the world. He was a distant relative of James Dean and looked it too, with his hair falling to the side and all-American handsomeness.

Like Pavlov's dog, I was a sucker for seasonal marketing. Now that fall was in full force, it seemed every store had some kind of pumpkin something. Pumpkin lattes. Pumpkin scones. Pumpkin donuts. Pumpkin cream cheese.

I loved them all. But I had a secret. I had already sampled most of those things within a week after Labor Day, even when it was eighty degrees and still feeling summery. I would escape from my desk, from my life, to try to eat away what was stressing me out: the laundry pile that never got smaller, the job search that never ended, the preschool bills that kept getting bigger.

I'd stuff it down bite by bite—that I wasn't working, that I felt fat. That every day I wanted to crush my weight problem, only to be crushed by it. I was unemployed, laid off after a decade of being a newspaper reporter.

Like a whistle drowning out everything that was on my mind, it was a noise so loud it drowned out the chaos. I needed to drown out the voice that told me I was a big pile of shit. That I was never going to find a job. That I was not worthy of being a wife to someone so wonderful. That I was a terrible mother. That everything I started would end in failure, especially diets.

I love my husband. He met me at my heaviest but still loved me, first as a friend for a decade and then as a wife. But I sometimes felt as if I were having an affair. Except instead of the proverbial lipstick on my collar, I had crumbs on my sweaters. I'd brush them off, praying that Chris wouldn't check the credit card bill and notice my string of purchases at fast food joints and bakeries. Mostly, I paid in cash.

With him, I pretended to have it all under control. That's because he's the most balanced person I know. To him, food is just food.

Since we were just running out for breakfast, I didn't feel the need to change. I was known around town for wearing sweatpants. I would spend the day in them with the intention of working out at some point, only to fall asleep in them later. Sneakers were the only shoes that were comfortable under my girth.

As we headed out, I didn't tell him that I'd already inhaled two iced-pumpkin scones (at almost 500 calories each) earlier that week while waiting for the barista to hand me my coffee (which, by the way, had a dollop of whipped cream on top). Instead, that morning with my husband, while he ordered his donut, I perked myself up and said, "I'll have the egg white sandwich."

As I gnawed through the floppy, overcooked egg circle smashed between two cardboard-like pieces of flatbread, I tried to figure out what the squares of red and green were in the egg. Perhaps they were green and red peppers. Certainly that counted as a serving of vegetables.

I thought how much more I would have enjoyed those scones if I'd eaten them with my husband sitting across the table. I wouldn't be as heavy if I just indulged once a week or so when I was with Chris, I thought to myself.

My daughter blissfully munched on her pumpkin donut. I hoped she'd know nothing of this—this mind game that consumed me morning to night.

At that point, Chris and I could have used some more early-morning togetherness. Ever since our daughter was born, we were too tired for our pre-parenthood morning ritual of coffee and conversation. Worse, with the extra weight on my frame, I worried that one day my husband might go to work and not return. Each night, I was surprised to see him walk through the door.

When we occasionally went out on a date, I didn't like dressing up. I wore the same jeans with the worn-through inner thighs when we went to the movies. My thighs flopped over the cup holders, making our giant Diet Coke and popcorn unstable.

My weight and eating habits had always been a touchy topic for us. Chris is an average-sized guy, content with three square meals a day and a snack. Mostly, he stayed mute on the subject, but once in a while, he'd venture a gentle "Should you be eating that?"

One birthday, he gave me a book about healthy eating, and I exploded. "Who buys a diet book for his wife on her birthday?!" No wonder he pretty much kept mum.

Like a hedgehog pudgy and spiky, I rolled into a ball to protect myself.

All my life I've avoided talking about my eating. But I needed someone to speak up, to bring my eating out into the open. I had been an unchecked closet eater for nearly three decades.

MY PARENTS CERTAINLY DIDN'T SAY anything when my eating problem started. It must have sounded like a mouse in the closet. Nine-year-old fingers scratching, pulling, peeling at a can in the dark.

I was in the pantry. My parents, still together at the time, were in the kitchen fighting. They didn't know I had snuck in there. Not that it mattered. I don't remember what they were fighting about. It was in the months before their separation. I was too occupied to pay attention to their words. While they each have their own stories about why they split, I was in the dark room, alone, ignoring it all.

I remember thinking I had to get into that can. I had seen it earlier when my mother unloaded groceries. On the outside of the small cylinder were pictures of bakery-perfect pastries. I wanted to eat all of them. I pulled off the plastic lid and tried to lift the metal tab. I gave it a solid yank, creating a ripping sound. My mother cracked open the door. There

I was caught with the can. I was afraid I'd be punished, a spin-off of the rage they felt toward each other.

I looked down, filled with the shock and disappointment of getting caught. "Nuts!"

In the light, I realized that I had just opened a can of walnuts. I realized the pictures of all those confections were what one could make with walnuts, not what one could immediately pop in her mouth upon opening the can.

My parents seemed angry that I had raided the pantry. I was mad that I hadn't found brownies.

After that, there would be many more instances, both in and out of the pantry, to come. I would get sneakier and quieter over the years. My fingers grew deft at pulling confections out of packages without a single crinkle of the surrounding wrapper. I could hold food in my cheek like a hamster, masterfully chewing without making a sound.

Eating had saved me, or so I thought. It would later save me from disappointments and trauma for years to come.

But every now and then, when I was eating healthily, I'd have a moment of clarity that food was indeed killing me. Food lifted me out of my world, but then it suffocated all that I wanted to be. Draining the enjoyment from family meals, and preventing me from activities I enjoyed.

Back at home after breakfast with my family, after the gnarly egg sandwich, I knew I wanted something else, not only to eat but out of life. I returned to my desk and saw my certificate from my first Kilimanjaro climb on the wall to the right of my desk, hanging with my other accolades next to my vision board. The absence of any kind of award from the second attempt was glaring. Sometimes I felt like taking the certificate down because every time I saw it, it reminded me that I didn't make it the next time. I knew I wanted to be back to where I had been physically and emotionally during that first climb.

I wanted to return to Kilimanjaro, to finish on top, but I could barely get outside for walks. I had all the time in the world, a daughter in full-time preschool, and I couldn't get it together.

Somehow I ended up in a shouting match with my brain about all the things I needed to do: look for a job, take a shower, clean the house, exercise.

I couldn't find the right order so nothing got done.

I couldn't look for a job until I took a shower.

I couldn't shower until I exercised.

I couldn't exercise until I cleaned the house.

If I cleaned the house there would be no time to look for a job.

I stood in my own way, rustling through the cabinets, eating away the shame of not getting anything done. Adding more shame to my plate about eating instead of accomplishing.

That was my daily to-do list. Eat. Cover the tracks.

WE HAVE TO EAT TO live. But I was living to eat. Deep inside I wanted to run away from myself, from this constant back and forth with food. I wanted to be normal. I wanted food to just be food. But sometimes, I worried I was too far gone.

The mail had come while we were at breakfast. I reached into the rusting metal box, worried about what bills I'd have in my hand. There was an REI photo postcard featuring a hiker somewhere amazing. It was a beautiful soft peach vista on a mountaintop. She looked healthy, happy, and in control.

I held the postcard in my hand, looking at it while fumbling with the lock to our condo, and thought, I just want to be there.

Whatever my weight, there was something about a travel adventure catalogue that made some part of me come alive. I would flip through glossy photos of Machu Picchu, the Alps, and other exotic locations, picturing myself doing all the things I loved. All the while devouring a king-size Kit Kat bar, chewing away my ambition, solidifying the shame of my current state. That was what inspired my first Kilimanjaro climb.

Something inside of me wanted to be a hiker girl, the kind who wore cute Patagonia fleece jackets and toted around a Nalgene water bottle. Instead, I walked around with a cup of coffee loaded with cream and sugar to ramp up between sugary snacks.

I kept telling myself that I would go on those adventure trips when I lost weight. I would get that sporty fleece jacket when it fit. But then I never lost weight. As age thirty approached, something clicked. I decided that I needed to stop being a victim of my fate (or my weight). The longer I put off pursuing my dreams, the harder they would be to achieve. So on New Year's Eve of 2005, I decided to stop tethering my life to the scale. I was ready to be free. Instead of going from diet to diet, I vowed to look at weight loss as a lifelong journey. I didn't want to keep putting things off anymore.

That year, instead of scrawling a resolution about how many pounds I wanted to lose (my New Year tradition), I wrote that I wanted to hike mountains. That resolution eventually led to my losing 120 pounds and completing my first trek up Mount Kilimanjaro.

I felt like I had two identities. The first was this woman who couldn't control her eating and was constantly trying to prove that she had worth by showing up at Weight Watchers meetings and exercising. Then she would show she was a complete and total failure by getting in line at the bakery.

Then there was the hiker girl—a bit like the REI model. She was always toting a Nalgene bottle, always ready for an adventure. She might even like kale.

I had covered the hiker girl, buried her under my own body weight. She was nearly dead.

It was time to revive her. Going back to Kilimanjaro for a third time felt like the only way to do so. The only choice was to go up.

CHAPTER 4

Bear Mountains

NEW YORK AND CONNECTICUT, 2010

I GOT AN E-MAIL FROM Sally, a Washington correspondent I had met at
The Weight of the Nation, a Centers for Disease Control and Prevention
event about obesity. I wanted her to do a story on my first climb and
weight loss in 2008. I was so proud of the accomplishment of losing 120
pounds. I wanted the world to know.

She never did that story, but in her e-mail she told me I had been on
her mind over the past couple of years. We were on opposite ends of the
size spectrum. I was six feet tall and fat. Sally was four feet, eleven inches,
and slender. For more than four decades, people had underestimated her
because of her size. They thought she was too tiny to participate in ath-
letics, too small to get the biggest stories at work, and too small to mind
being teased for being little. Still, she wanted to do big things.

Kilimanjaro was one of the items on her bucket list, but it was such
a huge mountain that it always intimidated her. After she met me, she
thought, "If she can do it, I can do it."

And, if she was going to climb Kilimanjaro, she wanted it to be
with me. But when Sally e-mailed me in 2011, I wasn't the 240-pound
version of myself she had met a few years back.

She said she wanted to bring her friend and fellow triathlete Tracey along for the journey. They vowed to raise a dollar per foot climbed—19,343 feet.

The invitation was my opening to have one more shot on the mountain. I knew, in addition to helping them reach their goal, I could raise another $5,000 for AIDS orphans and erase the memory of my second attempt by finishing on top. I just couldn't leave that much money on the table for Global Alliance for Africa.

Sally and Tracey thought of the mountain as a stepping-stone to celebrate Sally's fiftieth birthday and help them both train for the IRON-MAN Arizona, better known as IMAZ. An IRONMAN Triathlon is a 2.4-mile swim, a 112-mile bike ride, and a 26.2-mile run (or marathon) to cap it off, all done within a seventeen-hour window.

I immediately admired their "get-it-done" attitude. Tracey set up a website, listing their ambitions and calling on the supportive community of Team Z, a triathlete group in Washington, D.C., to rally behind them. Sally and Tracey set up raffles, cocktail parties, and a social media campaign to reach their financial goal.

They set up camping and hiking adventures to prepare for the hike because, well, Sally had never actually camped as an adult and had just committed to spending a week in the wild. Tracey taught Sally to start a fire, pitch a tent, and then break camp down. Even though all that stuff would be taken care of on the mountain by porters and guides, they wanted to be prepared. It was just their way. They even made a video of breaking down camp. Sally practiced rolling up a sleeping pad, and giggled her way through stuffing a sleeping bag into its sheath and collapsing tent poles. Sally celebrated each accomplishment by doing a little happy dance or reaching her arms up to the sky as if she'd crossed a finish line.

Normally, this sort of athlete—the kind who would take on swimming, biking, and running in one event, with shorts that exposed her rippling thigh muscles—intimidated me. This sort of athlete had perfect matching tops and bottoms, typically accented in turquoise, hot pink, chartreuse, or all three. This sort of athlete could talk for hours about detoxes, energy drinks, and interval training. Did I want to go with them for a week while hauling my flabby ass up the mountain?

I decided to meet them for a training hike to be sure I could stand them. We decided on Bear Mountain State Park, New York, a trek straight up that joins the Appalachian Trail. We chose the spot because my daughter was coming along for the hike, and there's a lovely merry-go-round at the bottom.

Unlike the steep trail, I found Sally and Tracey easygoing and gentle. Both were set for adventure. Sally wore a sky-blue button-down microfiber shirt and zip-off pants. Tracy pulled her brown shoulder-length hair into a ponytail and wore a coral shirt and khaki pants. They looked like hikers.

After our introductions and handshakes, Tracey announced, "We're back-of-the-pack triathletes. We pull up the rear."

In other words, they finished, but they often finished last. But to them, the important thing was they finished together. At races, theirs was often the last car in the parking lot. I liked that about them. They were slow like me.

Sally had a longtime boyfriend and Tracey was married. Neither had children but they took care of each other.

Tracey brought Nutella for a snack. I looked longingly at the velvety hazelnut spread and wished I had brought some too. But I knew I could never have Nutella in my home. I thought about every which way to use it—putting it on my toast, dunking some in my coffee, and licking it right from a spoon. Tracey, however, wasn't heavy like me. She couldn't be. Their weekly IMAZ workouts included two predawn one-hour swim practices, two speed or hill workouts on a bike, a long distance ride, two running group meets, and one long distance run on the weekends.

During all this, Tracey also found time to endure grueling physical therapy appointments to overcome a chronic knee ailment that could have prevented her from taking on the mountain. She suffered through shots to numb and lubricate the joint and pushed through it all.

By the end of the hike with Sally and Tracey, my daughter Anna had ripped her pants on a rock and was walking down the mountain without pants, wearing my jacket as a skirt. They took it in stride.

I decided I could live with them on Kilimanjaro for a week.

A FEW WEEKS AFTER THE hike with Sally and Tracey, the leaves started to turn brilliant yellow, red, and orange. Stacey, my husband's cousin, who was about one hundred pounds overweight, called me wanting to meet up for a hike.

"So, do you have room for one more?" she asked about the climb that she knew I was planning. She had wanted to join me in my second climb, but her finances were unraveling at the time. Ultimately, I was glad she didn't join because of my failure. Stacey had lost both parents within two years and had spent the past seven years eating and shopping. Now she wanted (or needed) an adventure to focus her attention on something else.

She thought things were tough when her mother died of cancer in late 2002. Then two years later, her father, my husband's uncle, was stabbed to death in Moab, Utah, on Mother's Day while trying to help a stranded motorist. He didn't know the motorist was craving methamphetamines.

I was engaged to Chris when I met Stacey at her father's funeral. She was quite thin then, but I didn't know anything else about her. I suppose I wanted to know her, but at the time I couldn't move beyond just feeling so terribly sad.

I could only say, "Are you okay?" or "Can I get you anything?" so many times before it was annoying. I wished I had something to say but I didn't know her father, only that he was an outdoorsman who was well loved by his family. He was an admired adventurer.

I let the cousins take over the conversation in the church reception as I munched on a sandwich made from meat from the platter of cold cuts and white bread.

In the years since then, as she put on the pounds, we had more in common.

After her father's death, Stacey couldn't sleep without Ambien, a prescription sleep aid. Even with two Labrador dogs—one yellow and one black—she felt afraid in her own home, just outside of Boston. She would check every lock and window before settling down for the night. In the same year, she divorced her husband and lost both her maternal and paternal grandmothers. Eventually, she had to give up her home as her debts exceeded her income and she went through both parents' estates.

She was nervous, of course, about taking this journey but felt very strongly that this was something she must do.

We decided to meet to hike Connecticut's highest peak, which also happened to be named Bear Mountain. We took the long way to get there, eight miles over many mountaintops to the 2,316-foot summit, and returned to the cars at the trailhead only at dusk.

I liked hiking with her because we were family, and on Kilimanjaro she would be someone on my team to balance out Sally and Tracey, who already knew each other well. But also, it felt nice having someone along who was also plus-sized. I figured with two of us on the mountain, even if she wasn't nearly my size, I wouldn't look so odd.

With Stacey's commitment to raise another $5,000 and Sally and Tracey's commitment to raise $20,000, we were on the line to raise nearly $30,000 for AIDS orphans, a monumental amount for Global Alliance for Africa. Supporting AIDS orphans is a cause I fell in love with after U2 front man Bono so valiantly spoke out about the scourge of AIDS in sub-Saharan Africa.

Supporting these kids and trying to make their childhoods better was something that felt very important to me. I wanted them to feel nurtured, to feel loved.

But from a more selfish point of view, something about putting myself out there as an adventurer made me feel good about myself. Raising money made me feel worthwhile as a human being, as if I was announcing to the world, "I don't just sit around. I work out. I can climb to the top of the tallest mountain in Africa even though I crumble at the sight of a cupcake."

You know, not all fat people are lazy.

While pledges for my trek totaled around $5,000, the tone of the people wishing me adieu was different from that for the first or even the second climb, when people were saying "You go, girl!" and "I'm so proud of you."

People knew I had gained the weight back. Many people turned down a donation this time around even though they had given in the past. I couldn't help but think this cause didn't make their list of contributions this time around because I was so heavy.

"We're all saying a little prayer," my upstairs neighbor said.

"You're so brave," said my yoga teacher, Reina.

I knew this time I needed to train, unlike my last failed trip. I needed to work as hard as I could physically, even if I didn't eat right.

I knew with my extra pounds, reaching the summit could very well be out of reach. I intended to drop fifty pounds during the six months I'd spend training for this climb. I spent weekends on the trails of New Jersey and weekdays on a spinning bike and treadmill. In fact, weight loss was one of the main reasons I'd decided to put myself through this hell a third time. Some people go on diets. I climb mountains.

Paleo, South Beach, or even Weight Watchers felt far more intimidating than Kilimanjaro.

Truthfully, with my struggle with food, hiking is probably the only thing that kept me from keeling over. However, if I was going to hike all the way up Kilimanjaro again, a week of grueling trekking to the top of Africa's highest peak, I'd have to go deep and leave it all on the mountain.

CHAPTER 5

Working It Out

SUMMIT, NJ, 2011, TWO MONTHS BEFORE THE THIRD CLIMB

I FELT EVERY BLADE OF grass, every pebble below the palms of my hands, as I extended my body into a plank in Bryant Park, a recreational area in my hometown of Summit, New Jersey.

My personal trainer was Heather Worthy, a short, muscle-bound woman who had spent much of her career as the trainer for Seton Hall University's men's basketball team, and most of her days in spandex. She unrolled a rope ladder, and it was my job to travel through it on my hands in plank position. It shouldn't have been much of a surprise; it was something she'd been making me do since spring. The grass was dryer and bristly but I was stronger.

When I started training three months before on a damp spring day, I could only make it through two squares before collapsing. I thought of that as I saw the rope extended across the park, people running around a paved walking path, staring at me as if I was the center ring entertainment.

Heather had taken me on as a charity project. I didn't have the money for a personal trainer, but I needed someone to inspire me to work harder. It was her. Her voice was husky, the kind you didn't want to defy, especially because she brought boxing gloves for the workout.

"All the way down," Heather said, instructing me to straighten my body into a plank. Sweat dripped off my brow and was immediately absorbed by the ground below.

I grunted, stepped my feet back, and started to move my hands from square to square, letting my feet follow.

"I'm low," I said, taking a whiff of the dry grass.

"Lower," Heather said.

I stepped my feet back so I could press my hands on the ground, feeling a tug in my core somewhere below my layers of fat, holding my whole body together. I tried to sink my body down into a straight line, like a bench, parallel to the ground. It came to my attention that I didn't like the plank position one bit. I thudded through each loop—eighteen in all—and nearly wept at the end. I had done it. My biceps and shoulders burned. I took in the accomplishment, sat on my heels, and prayed that would be it for the day.

While I wasn't going anywhere requiring ladders or ice axes, just this simple task of crossing the ladder showed me I was getting stronger.

"Alright, it's time for burpees," she said. I was forced to stand up, and got right into it, plunking my hands on the ground, kicking my legs out into a plank, and then hopping, maybe more like stumbling, my way back again.

"One," she counted. "We're doing fifteen."

Fuck off, I thought. Thank you was what I meant.

I was determined to make it up the mountain, no matter where I was on the scale. That meant getting stronger, building from the inside out. That meant becoming a gym rat again, just as I had been on my first trek up Kilimanjaro. Heather would lead me into the Summit YMCA weight room, which was stacked with buff and beautiful people, and make me bench press. My flab dangled off both sides of the weight bench. I wasn't lifting anything but the bar, but the mere fact of being in the room with others who were in good shape made me feel like I was something, or rather someone, special.

In the mirror, I would sometimes catch someone staring at me—typically a perfect, Lululemon-clad woman or a buff guy spotting another muscle-bound guy at the bench presses—and they'd immediately look down. Busted, I thought.

While others still saw me as fat, my hips felt more firm than flabby. My tummy was a little tighter. When I sucked it in, it actually moved. Working out was working out.

I made training a priority. I took yoga as often as I could with Reina, an instructor who inspired me to fold myself over "like a grilled cheese sandwich" to touch my toes, and got me into poses I couldn't believe I could do.

I hiked on my birthday. I hiked on the weekdays. One day, to prove how much better I'd feel after taking twenty pounds off my body, I suited up with twenty pounds of sugar in my backpack.

As my boots and I hiked up the first steps of Mount Tammany, I saw a yellow sign. "Warning: Copperhead and Rattle Snake habitat."

The snakes liked to live in the rocks that made the hill. Those rocks were what I needed to climb. This steady hand-over-hand trek was the perfect training exercise for Jamaica Rocks, the last leg of Kilimanjaro. "I hope they don't like sugar," I said to my hiking companion, Jen, who also lived in Summit. Jen wanted to take on Kilimanjaro eventually but was really just passing the time after more than a year of unemployment, one of the many financial folks out of work after the 2008 financial crisis. She had explained what she did for work once, but I stopped understanding it when it came to numbers. Either way, she wanted something else to focus on, so we hiked.

I was glad I found her. She was someone to be accountable to and meet for training hikes. I couldn't blow off my training with her.

She said she was glad she found me, since being outside was a good break from constantly checking LinkedIn. Also it gave her a chance to talk through her latest job interview drama. Potential employers would tell her she was a perfect fit for an open position but never call her back. She had to go through demeaning numerical tests when she had been a financial professional for two decades. She felt vulnerable, and walking up a mountain with me made her feel strong.

For our Mount Tammany training trek, I suited up in a pink shirt and black athletic capris made out of a kind of polyester. Juxtaposed with my SmartWool hiking socks and boots, it didn't look right. I never looked right, I thought as I clunked along, dragging my red Swiss Army hiking poles up the trail, which was secured by railroad ties.

As we stepped into the forest, the rocks seemed to glow with moisture and lichen. The Delaware River runs next to these woods separating New Jersey and Pennsylvania, along with Route 80. Sometimes it was hard to tell if you were hearing the rustle of the highway or the water.

The first mile of the trail was nothing but up. I'd step to the side and have to catch myself from toppling over because of the extra weight in my backpack. Even if I didn't drop twenty more pounds, I proved to myself that I didn't want to be burdened with any more weight. I had more than I could handle.

We passed a few hikers who gave me that "I'm so glad you're hiking, but please don't die" look.

I sometimes wish other people would do this: put on a heavy pack so they could feel what it was like to actually walk in my shoes. I wished people who teased me had to wear the fat suit Gwyneth Paltrow wore while filming *Shallow Hal*, and try walking down the block. If they made it that far, then they could try taking a hike.

My backpack wobbled back and forth with each step—like a wriggly child on my back trying to switch sides to get a better view. The sugar made it very unstable and difficult to manage.

Jen was kind and waited at the top of each pass for me. Her perfectly blond hair was pulled back in a ponytail and she wore shorts fit for tennis or hiking. My hair matted to my forehead with sweat. I'd stop whenever possible and lift my chartreuse Nalgene bottle to my lips.

We wound through the woods that smelled of rich earth and moss, making our way to a viewpoint to let others on the path pass so they didn't have to veer onto the sprouting forest off trail. I admired the white mountain laurel blossoms just to catch a break. I stood, hands on my hips with my backpack tugging at my shoulders, wondering how much longer this would take.

I strained and sweated as lean hikers passed me by carrying nothing but a water bottle. I leaned into the rocks, letting them hold me and using them as a launching pad for the next step. And the next. I made it to the top that day. I was sweaty and sore—especially my shoulders where my backpack straps tugged at me—but I made it.

I did this over and over in woods throughout New Jersey. I took long slogs wherever I could, hugging the shoulder of New Jersey roads to places like the Watchung Reservation, a 1,945-acre wood in the middle of suburban New Jersey.

I found myself fumbling through the medicine cabinet searching for ibuprofen after these hikes. The pain reliever was among all the other things I had there to quell the symptoms of obesity: antacids for heartburn and baby powder for chafing legs.

The ibuprofen pills rattled as I tried to open the white childproof top. I poured the brownish orange pills on my hand; after the sugar hike, I was in need of three to silence my barking back. I placed them on my tongue, cupped water from the faucet into my hands, and slurped them down. After ten miles of hiking, I didn't want to have to saunter down the hallway of our one-floor condo to the kitchen for a glass.

As I stretched out my legs in bed, I let out a bellowing "Ahhh."

My feet were raw. My thighs were chafed. There was such sweet relief in being horizontal, being free of carrying myself.

When my husband came in, I rolled over hoping he didn't want sex. I was just spent. I let my hands drift down below my waistline. I clutched the pouch of fat that had cascaded six inches below my belly since college.

It was loose, jiggly, as if my bag was emptying. Still, I was 3X and I felt like I was thirty-seven going on seventy years old.

The number on the scale didn't descend much below 290. But I was building strength. I was losing fat. I was a linebacker.

CHAPTER 6

Mad Marathon

SUMMIT, NJ, AND WAITSFIELD, VT, 2011,
ONE MONTH BEFORE MY THIRD CLIMB

In the doctor's office, waiting for a shot, I felt a cold pall wash over me as I had so many times when I was a kid. I didn't even like to swallow pills. My mother had to crush them between two spoons and add them to a teaspoon of strawberry jelly.

However, a trip to Africa comes with a lot of prescriptions. Dr. Mendiola, a travel medicine specialist, seemed excited about the number of things he could dole out for one journey to Kenya and Tanzania. He handed me four little blue squares of paper with prescriptions:

- *Malarone to prevent malaria*
- *Ambien so I could sleep on the plane*
- *Ciprofloxacin in case I suffered severe diarrhea that even Imodium couldn't stop*
- *Dexamethasone to quell altitude sickness. (Most people are given Diamox, but as it's a sulfa drug I'm allergic.)*

But before I left, there was one more thing: a typhoid fever shot.

I couldn't escape out the window. I was far too big for the shoe-box-sized opening. I reminded myself that I needed this immunization to survive as he came in with a dose of typhoid vaccine and a syringe. Typhoid causes a red, spotty rash, a high fever, hallucinations, encephalitis, hemorrhaging in the intestines, enlarging of the spleen and liver. And I was allowing him to inject me with it?

I need this to be well, I told myself again and again. In a quick pinch, it was over, and I was on my way home. Like most things I worry about, it wasn't nearly as bad as I had imagined.

Later that week, I went for a general health checkup from Dr. Meyer, a spritely being who had been my doctor for years. While she presented my physical results to me, my calves and feet dangled from the exam table like two logs about to teeter off a waterfall. Blood pressure, blood sugar, and cholesterol: all perfect.

I was always surprised to hear that.

Dr. Meyer, who was lean, with short brown hair, admired my climbs over the years because she believed exercise kept my insides healthy. So did I.

Still, for years, I'd come out of doctor's visits shocked I wasn't diagnosed with diabetes from all the sugar I ate. As an obese person, it felt like I was supposed to be really sick, a goner. Excess weight was supposed to be a prescription for diabetes, for cancer, for heart disease. I had none of those things. With all my physical activity, it felt like I was cheating the system.

"Many of my overweight patients who exercise are in much better shape than the skinny ones who don't," said Dr. Meyer. But the visit wasn't all smiles and congratulations.

"Your BMI comes out to forty," she said, looking at the screen. "You're in the danger zone for long-term complications. It won't be long before you start feeling it in your joints."

She was right. My hip had been nagging me. I felt a pinching feeling as I walked. I didn't want to say anything. I hoped it would heal itself somewhere between here and Africa. I had a lot more hiking to do.

I had to keep moving. I had to keep being active. I feared that I was one workout from not being able to do any of it. Like I was a few steps away from needing a walker. A cane. Orthopedic shoes. So much of my life was spent being almost handicapped, with a handicap that I created. I was the one who fueled the impending immobility with my eating. Yet, somewhere inside of me, I wanted to fight back.

Even though I was having success with training, I was still struggling with food. Up until the month before I left for Kilimanjaro, the only times I wasn't eating were when I was at my computer typing away at job queries, looking for donations on behalf of my climb, at the gym, or when my family was around.

In between job inquiries, I found myself circling back to the fridge and cabinets. Like a cow in a pasture, I was in a constant graze. Digging my fingers into the shredded wheat box, polishing off a box of cereal bars the day after I picked them up from the store.

One time, I opened the freezer, and with the cold door against my back, I ate directly from a half gallon of ice cream. I returned there again and again, the spoon scraping against the side until it was empty and I was nowhere near full. I dashed to the store to replace it. As I was nearing the checkout, I ran into my husband's friend, who started chatting with me. I held the basket behind my leg, hoping he wouldn't see inside and mention it to Chris.

I stumbled through the conversation, still trying to hide the half gallon of ice cream with a cereal box, in case he came behind me to pay. I wanted it shoved in a bag before anyone else saw it.

When I got home, I hid half of it in a Tupperware container in the back of the freezer, to make it look like I hadn't touched it. But by the time I left to pick up my daughter, I had nibbled at it so much it was gone. I had another entire half gallon in the afternoon.

I didn't want to share what was going on with my husband and his parents, all of whom were vehemently supportive of my adventure, clearing their schedules to make it happen. While I had gone down many weight-loss paths, from strict low-carb regimens to Weight Watchers, Chris never gave up on me the way I gave up on myself. Then again, we had a way of supporting each other's dreams.

When Chris ran his marathons, Anna and I were his cheering

squad. When he had to be rehydrated in the medical tent after a particularly hot and muggy 26.2 miles, I held his hand. I bought energy gels and Gatorade for his practice runs. He would run as far as he could from home, twenty-two miles in the final training days, and I would pick him up if he overestimated the mileage. I wasn't a runner, but I wanted to be able to keep up with him.

I needed one last challenge to prove I could make it up the mountain. Chris knew this, and wanted me to succeed.

A few weeks after the ice cream incident, Chris called out to me from his office. "Hey, let's do this Mad Half Marathon," he said, summoning me into his man cave of guitars, overflowing bookshelves, and running medals. "It goes right by where we got married."

I leaned in to look at his laptop. I said yes immediately, feeling well trained but wanting to prove to Chris and myself that I could take on the mountain. The course passed The Skinner Barn, the historic refinished building where Chris and I were married in a Quaker wedding ceremony seven years prior. We sat in silence in front of a hundred of our friends and family members in prayer until we stood ready to say our vows.

ON OUR WEDDING DAY, A soft rain fell, making the colors of Vermont fall pop from the mountains around us. I wore a $220 plus-size dress I picked up at the Filene's Basement sale. I wasn't a Vera Wang kind of bride. That super-expensive stuff wouldn't fit me anyway.

Our Ben & Jerry's ice cream wedding cake, topped with roses, was a mutual choice. In fact, it was one of the few things Chris wouldn't budge on as far as our wedding budget went. Our wedding was a mostly DIY affair. My bridesmaids helped me pull together bouquets of flowers for their clutches and for my own bouquet—russet-red roses that looked like the maple leaves changing outside. They were so happy I found love, and did anything to make the wedding run smoothly—from tying raffia around the maple syrup favors to switching the dance-mix CDs Chris made for the occasion.

THREE AND A HALF HOURS into walking the Mad Half Marathon, I passed The Skinner Barn. I half expected to see Chris, even though he had been past it two hours before me. My hips burned. I wanted to stop but the race clock was ticking—each step would take me closer to him. I hurried to reach him, galumphing my way toward the finish line, needing to be in his embrace and recapture the feeling of our wedding day.

Even before the race, I needed to use the bathroom, but I couldn't squeeze anything out. All along the course, I searched for a place to stop, but everywhere was too exposed. I didn't want to be seen by a passing walker or even the cows in the meadows. At one point, I shat my pants, but I didn't want to get further behind so I kept walking. Thirteen point one miles later, I was finished. It helped knowing that Chris would be waiting for me at the finish line.

"Now that was hilly. You're looking so strong," Chris said when I finally met him at the finish line. He hugged my sweaty body.

"Careful, I'm disgusting," I said. I went to a porta-potty to clean up my soiled britches. I tried to tell him of my accident without anyone hearing me.

After I cleaned up, he brought me some apple cider, water, and Ben & Jerry's ice cream.

"You're going to make it up the mountain," he said and smiled.

CHAPTER 7

Baggage

Anna hopped up and down on the bed, nearly tumbling over the neat piles of clothes and gear I was preparing for the forty-mile journey up Mount Kilimanjaro. The mountain is just two hundred miles from the Equator, and yet the trek to the 19,343-foot peak would end near some of the world's fastest-melting glaciers. In other words, I needed to prepare for high heat and frigid cold. I needed to pack everything.

The gear covered my king-size bed, and it all had to be stuffed into one duffle bag, which grew smaller every time I added more items from the list.

Each time Anna jumped, all the gear—hydration pack tubing, glove liners—jumped with her, threatening to cascade over the edge. Inevitably, Anna plopped down in the middle of it all, causing a supply avalanche in my already messy bedroom, with dirty clothes and mismatched shoes strewn everywhere. As I started restacking, she got up and continued her jumping.

"Kili-ma-jaro. Kili-ma-jaro. Kili-ma-jaro," she chanted in her sweetest three-year-old voice. She knew Kilimanjaro was a big mountain. She could point to it on the globe. She knew I was going to hike it. She didn't know that there was a chance I wouldn't return.

About twenty-five thousand people attempt Kilimanjaro's summit each year. Only 66 percent make it to the top. About eight people a year die trying. None were as fat as me.

Just by being above the cloud line, I would be at risk for altitude sickness, which meant certain death for some climbers. Headache, nausea, and other stomach ailments were all par for the course. The real danger was pulmonary edema: the buildup of fluid in the lungs, causing a hiker to cough up froth and blood, leading to lung collapse and death. There was also the risk of cerebral edema: excess fluid in the brain that could lead to disorientation, madness, coma, and, yes, death. A permanent vacation.

That's not to mention the other dangers of being out in the open for eight days. Gnarly stomach bugs from soiled water or spoiled food. Twisted ankles, broken bones, and other injuries were all possible. So was a tumble off the trail, down thousands of feet, and off a rocky cliff. Then there were potential mudslides and the possibility of frostbite and hypothermia from a minus-twenty-degree cold snap.

Why was I doing this again?

To look at me, you wouldn't think I had a penchant for living dangerously. Or maybe you would? After all, at my weight, I was already at higher risk for diabetes, heart disease, cancer—you name it.

Of course, the biggest and most constant threat to my well-being was the high probability of my suffocating while ducking into the kitchen and stuffing something into my mouth, or shoving a stash of candy in my craw between red lights on my morning commute.

If someone happened to see me mid-binge, if they happened to come around the corner unexpectedly—my husband or even my three-year-old daughter—I could carry out a full conversation while hiding food. It was a truly ridiculous talent.

I was less adept at this packing thing. Altogether, the items on the two-page Kilimanjaro packing list could weigh no more than thirty-five pounds. That's because a porter would carry my gear up the mountain on his head. At first, I felt guilty that the only thing I would have to carry was a daypack stuffed with three liters of water, rain gear, and snacks. But in high-altitude hiking, where the trek becomes more arduous with each step toward the summit, even a daypack is a heavy load to bear.

My biggest challenge was that my clothes were bigger than the average hiker's. Just as I had on my last Kilimanjaro attempt, I was wearing hiking pants that were made from two single pairs sewn together. I couldn't even consider wearing the ultra-lightweight stuff at REI because it was mostly for "ultra-light" people. Instead, I bought my pants at Junonia, a plus-size active wear store. Even my sleeping bag was super-sized so it would zip over my hips. Three times as big as most sleeping bags, it came in a chunky, yellow nylon sheath and took up a third of my duffle bag. The bigger bag was lower-grade, the only thing I could find in the right size, meaning it might not be adequate protection against the subzero temperatures on the mountain. I would have to sleep in my long underwear, which barely fit over my bottom. I was going to have a very cold butt crack, which I worried would also peek out of my ill-fitting pants.

Then again, nothing ever fit with me. When my grandmother Margaret was alive, she bought my winter coats, trying to take that expense from my single mother, who worked the evening shift as a nurse to support my brothers and me. I loved flipping through the Sears or JC Penney catalogues in my grandma's overheated senior apartment, dreaming of what I could buy.

I wanted wool peacoats like the cool kids, but I often couldn't find a size that would fit. I figured I could leave the coat open, that one day I'd diet down enough that it would button up over my hips. She bought me what I wanted, hoping it would help me fit in even if it didn't fit me.

Before bedtime, she'd ask me to dish out ice cream for the two of us before tucking me in on her pullout couch. Her afghan was lumpy. The metal bars of the bed jutted into my back. When she couldn't walk, I'd go across the street to Kerry's convenience store to pick up cans of Hormel chili to supplement her Meals on Wheels food. Once in a while when she was feeling adventurous, we'd take the walker across the street and sit down to have meatball sandwiches together. It was one of the few times I went to restaurants as a kid. Maybe clothes would never fit me, and I would never fit in at school, but I did fit here. But with my grandmother, I felt at home. I felt love. I felt warmth.

UNLIKE IN ELEMENTARY SCHOOL, ON Kilimanjaro, my jacket had to close. I had to be warm and dry to ensure my safety. But because of my size, I had to omit some things from the packing list: rain pants (there were none in my size) and gaiters (none fit around my calves). If there was a torrential downpour, I would be soaked and miserable, not to mention freezing, for the remainder of the trip.

The plan was to sort the clothes according to the days I would wear them, then stuff them into large Ziploc bags. An experienced hiker had given me this tip. This would keep the items dry no matter what the weather turned out to be. Plus, hikers tend to get a bit loopy above the cloud line, so it was best to have each day's items sorted and ready.

This system would also help me keep up with the schedule. No morning searches for socks and clean underwear. I'd need that time to wrestle my gargantuan sleeping bag into its yellow sleeve. My daughter had used a permanent marker to draw a stick figure of me on the mountain on each Ziploc bag. The last one was with my arms outstretched on the top. The bubble head had a big smiley face on it.

"That's the day," I told Anna, "I will start coming down the mountain and back to you."

Thinking again of the dangers, I started to second-guess my plans. I had to go. I didn't want to back out on myself. I'd spent my lifetime backing out. I avoided roller coasters for fear that I wouldn't fit in the safety harness or that my weight would send everyone crashing to their death. I avoided sitting on the floor with my daughter for fear that I wouldn't be able to get back up.

I watched my daughter, who was oblivious to my self-doubt, bouncing on the bed. Her blond hair, as straight as mine, floated skyward; her butterfly skirt puffed up with each bounce. I wondered what adventures were in store for her. I wondered if what I was doing would inspire her to take on big goals.

I also wondered if I would leave her motherless, and leave my husband a single parent. I was taking this trip to support children across the globe. But I also needed to be around to support my own child. I couldn't do that if I was dead: from the mountain or from obesity.

I want to return to her. I need to return to her. Maybe I shouldn't go?

I think of anything as an opportunity for weight loss. But, like most pound-shredding endeavors I've tried in my life—Weight Watchers, delivered meals, protein powders—this one failed. I lost a handful of pounds, but I needed to drop a butt-load more. I was out of time, just a few days from departure.

Despite my doubts, I couldn't bring myself to cancel the trip. As with my previous hikes up Kilimanjaro, my supposed goal was to raise money for AIDS orphans in Africa. Whatever my personal failures, the hike could still benefit others—or at least that was my reasoning. I needed to honor my commitments, model good behavior for Anna.

I wanted to prove to my daughter, to everyone, that I was capable of really living, of doing great things, even if I happened to be fat. It would be great if I could also prove to Anna, and the world, that I could eat like a normal person.

Baby steps, Kara. Baby steps.

I also wanted to stop being an embarrassment. Earlier in the year, when I'd visited Anna's preschool, one of her classmates started chanting, "Your butt is so big. You have a big butt."

I tried to hide behind the wooden play fridge, nearly knocking it over along with the fake ketchup bottles and wooden hot dogs. I was frozen, as if in a spotlight, finally being called out for who I was.

I needed to sign Anna in, but I wished I could have vanished on the spot.

I was familiar with the way kids latch on to things they want to talk about and won't let go. This was age three. Anything that was different was worth mentioning or, better yet, shouting about. But this boy, Tommy, with his adorable button eyes and straight-cut bangs, was relentless. He tried all ways of saying it.

"Mrs. Big Butt. Big, big butt. It is so gigantic."

First I wanted to smack the kid. I wanted to make him feel the sting of how I burned inside. But, of course, I knew that was not the right thing to do. I wanted to come back with a liberal, teachable moment, something better than a sheepish "People are all different sizes."

I didn't want to draw attention from the teacher. I didn't need another person in on this, knowing my torment. I was glad they were engrossed in craft projects with the other kids. But after a while, they couldn't ignore me looking like a bullfighter trying to cry for mercy from a raging animal.

"Now, be nice," I said, but I said it so weakly, so sheepishly, that he didn't hear me. I didn't want to engage other students. The boy kept chanting until a teacher admonished, "Now, that's not nice." I saw "I'm sorry" in the teacher's eyes.

I wanted to leave the room. I was mortified. Fortunately, my daughter had already made her way to the art table and didn't seem to hear the incident as she pasted colorful triangles to a paper, making a mosaic.

I tried to laugh it off. I looked away, wishing it hadn't happened, hoping it wouldn't happen again. I dreaded visiting her school for weeks after that. And if I did, I wore a big purple A-line raincoat to even out my lumps.

The ironic thing about being fat is that you don't want people to notice you, yet there you are, bigger than anyone. As if your body is screaming, "Notice me!" With every movement, every awkward lifting up out of a chair, you are undeniably noticeable. I wanted to hide, even at family parties. I inadvertently knocked coasters and picture frames off side tables with my hips constantly. Then, breathless from exertion and embarrassment, I bent to retrieve them, exposing my underpants and my giant rear.

I was sick of feeling so naked, as if I wore my issues on the outside. Earlier that year, I saw an overweight woman making her way through the grocery store in an electric scooter. She had swollen legs, a gargantuan neck, and jiggly arms. She filled her baskets with cupcakes and junk food. I wanted to look away. It looked like my possible future.

I wanted to get my weight under control before my daughter reached the cruelest age: middle school. But even if I didn't drop a pound, perhaps an achievement so great as hiking Kilimanjaro would stunt any embarrassment she had for me.

Still, what kind of mother would do something as dangerous as climbing a mountain at three hundred pounds? I decided to write my will before I left, and I also made Anna a construction-paper book bound with pipe cleaners. Worst-case scenario, I thought it would be something to remember me by. I called it "Mommy on the Mountain."

Mommy is traveling across the globe to conquer a mountain
   called Kilimanjaro.
The first few days will be a breeze as she walks by trees filled
   with monkeys.
Soon enough, she'll be above the clouds, blowing you kisses to where
   you are now.
She will start one last hike under the stars. All through the night.
   One step at a time, she'll be all right.
Then she'll reach the top, such a proud sight, after trying with all of
   her might.
A few more days and she'll head home, happy to be with her family
   who she loved all along.

I ROLLED UP MY HIKING pants to squeeze out the air (this would mean fewer wrinkles, not that it would matter after eight days without a shower) and watched Anna dance, twirl, and make a mess of my stuff. I didn't stop her, maybe because I felt guilty about leaving her. Finally, she hopped off the bed and stepped into a still-empty suitcase, plopping herself down.

"Mama, I want to come with you," she said. Her big blue eyes sought a yes.

I wished she could.

I should find a way, maybe a babysitter in Africa, so she can come along and then she can come on safari with me.

On second thought, did I really want a three-year-old along on a fourteen-hour-plus journey, not including travel connections, to Nairobi, Kenya? Especially a three-year-old who got carsick on the way to Target?

"No, sweetie. Not this time," I said. "You know you have to be ten years old to hike the mountain. How old are you?"

"Free-and-half," she said.

I was going to have enough tantrums of my own trying to make it up the mountain without giving my daughter a piggyback ride.

"It won't be long until you're old enough," I said, touching her hair. "You'll have so much fun when I'm gone. I can't wait to hear all about it."

I packed my beige Mad Half Marathon T-shirt to remind me of what I accomplished before Kilimanjaro. On the mountain, I wouldn't have Chris to take care of me after. I wasn't even sure I'd have cell service to let him know I was okay, or if I'd ended up going down the mountain in a wooden wheelbarrow with three bicycle wheels. Actually, that's if I was lucky. Most hikers who are evacuated from the peak have no choice but to hobble back down the same brutal terrain.

Last to go in my bag were what I thought of as the uncertainty supplies: duct tape, tampons (even if it wasn't that time of the month, the physical strain of the mountain could trigger my period), extra boot laces, a nail brush, and triple the amount of wet wipes that I thought I would need. I also packed two travel-size deodorants, wondering if they would make a difference with all the exertion.

I'd also prepared an energy bag stuffed with Clif Bars, sports gels, Emergen-C, and Airborne to temper the taste of the iodine tablets we'd be using to purify the water on our way up the mountain. We had to drink as many as five liters of water a day to guard against altitude sickness. Because of potential parasites, drinking it without iodine could be deadly. I also picked up coloring books and mini-boxes of crayons to give to kids along the lower portion of the trail. They liked to ask hikers for chocolate. At the last minute, I also decided to pick up some lollipops.

I stood in the Whole Foods "healthy" candy aisle, which was lined with lousy-tasting licorice and sesame candies, wondering if I should put the lollipops in my shopping cart. I took a step toward the shelf, then back, then decided to grab them. Supposedly they were organic, so how bad could they be? I tucked them deep down in my duffle bag so I wouldn't eat them myself on the way to the mountain. No candy is safe around me.

I pushed down on my bag, squeezing every last bit of air and volume out of everything so I could close the duffle bag. Slowly, my tower of fleece jackets settled into place. Straddling the bag, I pulled each side of the zipper together. It reminded me of desperately trying to close the fly on a pair of size thirty-two jeans at my peak weight of 360 pounds. And I'm not talking waist size. I'm talking the biggest number available at most plus-size stores.

I kneaded the bag like a cat, wedging in every last item until finally, I was able to pull the zipper up. Tooth by tooth I sealed the bag closed, like an overstuffed sausage. I was sure it exceeded the thirty-five-pound weight limit. I'd have to drop a few more items before the hike.

No, I told myself, that's not a reason to eat the lollipops before the trip.

CHAPTER 8

Squeezed

PLANE FROM AMSTERDAM TO NAIROBI

Everyone hated me the moment I stepped on the plane. Eyes bulged as they saw me thump down the jetway, with my daypack resting on the ridge of my rear. I knew what they were thinking: Please don't let her be seated next to me. I knew it because I've seen that look anytime I've gone anywhere on a plane. I'm not afraid of flying. I am afraid of airplane seats.

The average airplane seat is about eighteen inches across. Anyone with a more than thirty-six-inch hip circumference would feel squeezed. Mine was sixty-four inches.

I typically asked for an aisle seat so I could spill over into the middle. I'd move my leg out of the way when a beverage cart came through, but expect to be walloped a number of times throughout the trip. As always, at the gate, I asked if I could be moved to a place next to an empty seat, but this flight—KLM from Amsterdam to Nairobi, Kenya—was full.

As I stepped on the plane, I felt the jetway release under my girth. Sally, Tracey, and Stacey, whom I met in the Amsterdam airport, headed to their seats elsewhere on the plane. The flight attendant, who looked like Airplane Barbie with her tailored KLM outfit, looked me up and down and then pointed me to my seat.

"You're in Economy Plus," she said in an adorable Dutch accent and a little smile. "A little more legroom."

I gave her a big smile, as if trying to distract her from my size. "Going to be a long flight, eh?" I said, clutching my boarding pass. I cleared my throat and lowered my eyes and voice.

"When you have a minute, I'm going to need a seatbelt extender," I whispered.

I dreaded this moment, this ask. There was no way a regular seatbelt would fit around my waist. Airlines have seatbelt extenders, like the ones flight attendants use to demonstrate during plane safety. It's about three feet of extra belt, and a buckle that fastens to the regular band.

Most times, flight attendants are discreet, rolling the seatbelt extender up and holding it in the palm of their hands while walking through the plane. They find me (not that I'm easy to lose) and gently hand it your way. But in between the request and the delivery is the agony of wondering how it is going to be presented. I imagined a flight attendant shouting, "Now who was the large lady who needed this three feet of extra seatbelt?" There are always glances from fellow passengers, wondering what special thing I got from the attendant. So I fasten it quickly, hoping no one will notice that my seatbelt, when unbuckled, reaches the floor.

As the flight attendant went to search for the extra strap, I pretended I was diminutive, as I tried to sidestep through the plane, finding my way back to my seat. Even when people leaned in toward the windows, my hips smacked them in the shoulder and face as I passed. I knocked papers off tray tables. I tangled in their electronics cords. I felt like a hippo in a ballerina suit.

When someone tried to make his way up the aisle, there was an awkward, thou-shall-not-pass moment between the two of us. Eventually, he had to duck into another seat for me to clomp through.

I wasn't sure what was worse, getting to the seat first and seeing the person next to me arrive, acknowledging with a sigh that she has to sit next to me, or walking down the aisle and finding my row companion already situated, only to look me up and down with horror.

In this case, I arrived first.

I shifted the armrest up, hoping it would save me three inches. However, it made any audiovisual enjoyment impossible, since I couldn't see the volume controls. My headphone's wires were thrust into the sky, tangling me.

And then came the man with whom I would share these eight hours. He was a gray-haired businessman who looked like he was on his way to some kind of negotiation. He seemed to travel a lot. He probably had a number of things he didn't want to deal with on a plane. The roll of his eyes told me a fat row companion was at the top of his list.

"Hi there," I said as he sat down, immediately thrusting the armrest down on my hip, like a paper cutter blade on a stack of paper.

It was clear by the way he tucked away his things, and his grumbles underneath his breath, that he didn't want to know me. I was stuck on the inside of this row for eight hours.

What if I needed to go to the bathroom? But then again, I usually tried to avoid that if possible. That whole experience was its own adventure. Trying to fit in a closet, unfolding the door, while shimmying myself in to pee over a hole, the width of which was one-third the size of my ass.

I've always been a little awkward around men I don't know. I feel like I come across as desperate for affection, somehow just needing love. I wanted to flash my wedding ring, but remembered, I had left it home so the diamond—even if it was only a modest quarter carat my husband purchased in grad school—wouldn't get stolen in Africa or attract unnecessary attention to our group.

"I'm heading to Kilimanjaro to hike it for a third time," I announced to my neighbor, trying to cover for my girth. Really, I wanted to say, "I'm sorry for taking up so much space."

He gave me a "please stop talking" look and returned to his laptop.

In the tiny airplane seat, my rear stuck out five inches, as if I was wearing a pillow in my pants, which had the effect of pushing my knees into the seat back in front of me. I was stuck and had to stay that way, my eyes fixed on my tray table. Sometimes I jotted things down in my journal, pulling it out of the seat pocket in front of me where I had stored it before takeoff. But when I dropped my pen, I was stuck with just an in-flight magazine and the monitor in front of me.

I kept returning to the electronic map on the seat back in front of me that was tracking our progress, hoping time would speed up and the trip would be over quickly, like the travel scenes in *Indiana Jones— Raiders of the Lost Ark.*

The fifty-something graying guy next to me hated me, I thought, as the airplane droned on. I looked at the map again. No visible progress.

Waiting for the beverage or meal cart was my only entertainment. I watched the two flight attendants, working in tandem, go all the way up the aisle of the plane and waited painfully for them to work their way back.

When my Diet Coke finally came, I had to hold it, otherwise it would have slid right off my tray table into my neighbor's lap. I couldn't use my tray table because it wouldn't stay flat.

When it was time to rest, I just couldn't.

I had already watched two movies since takeoff, and we still had four hours to go. I felt every one of them, probably more than most people on the flight.

On airplanes, even mid-flight, I'm afraid of having a Kevin Smith moment. Kevin Smith is a filmmaker who was kicked off a Southwest Airlines flight for being too fat. Some heavy people need to buy two seats. In my case, I ordered a little extra legroom, but what I really needed was hip room.

I craned my neck to find Sally, Tracey, and Stacey in the rows behind me but couldn't see them. Good thing, I thought. We were going to be spending enough time together on the mountain. I didn't need to be squishing them on the airplane. I didn't want them to see how miserable I made the people next to me.

I tried to get my pen again, but my belly folded over and squeezed the air out of my lungs. I shifted my girth, but I couldn't reach it. I couldn't touch the ground. I didn't want to wake my already peeved neighbor, so I sat there with nothing to do but watch movies. When the meal came, I had to eat it fast, so it wouldn't slide down onto my knees.

"This is a lot of food," said the guy next to me. He had awakened briefly for his meal.

"Yeah." I took the wrapped dinner roll and stuck it in the front pocket and saved it for later. I hated those kinds of insertions as judgment about how fat I was. I wanted to make excuses, tell him my life story on this plane (we had time to do so), but instead I gave an impish nod. An admonishment for the way I was—and that maybe I should think about my weight.

Because I didn't have a parachute, I just had to sit through it. But I didn't want to listen to his judgments or anyone else's. A few minutes after the meal, the guy fell asleep again. I grabbed the dinner roll and gently unwrapped and ate it.

CHAPTER 9

Doing Good

NAIROBI, KENYA, A FEW DAYS BEFORE THE HIKE

I STOOD WITH MY NECK bent under the overhead compartment, just to let the blood return to my legs, breathing deeply the air that had been recycled on the plane for eight hours. Being cramped in an airplane seat for so long, I just needed to stand, even if it meant my rear and hips intruded on my neighbor.

After clumsily bonking into each seat on the way out of the aircraft, I rendezvoused with Sally, Tracey, and Stacey on the runway. The air smelled of city dust with a dense smattering of airplane fuel. All of us stumbled into the airport to find our way through Kenyan immigration and pick up our bags.

As the bags came out on a conveyor belt, a man approached me. He was tall, with a khaki baseball cap pushed down over his brow. I could see a paper sign printout in his hand, which read "Global Alliance for Africa."

"You must be Mama Kubwa," he said. The name was given to me during my first climb. It's Swahili for "big woman." Even at my skinniest—240 pounds—I was one of the largest women they had ever seen on

Kilimanjaro (they had plenty of men with beer guts on other climbs, but they didn't make a big deal about them).

I flung my fleece around my rear and tied it at my waist, but it stood out like a superhero cape.

The man introduced himself as Naiman. He stood, holding a clipboard, next to a trolley for our luggage. We lugged the cart to our van, piled the giant bags against the windows, and tied some of them to the roof. One bump on our way to the hotel would mean we'd be without everything. I realized that's why we were told to wear our hiking boots on the plane.

There was nothing truly fragile in my bags. I hadn't brought a laptop, though I felt empty to be without it. Being without my laptop reminded me of all the job searching I wasn't doing while on this trip. I'd been unemployed for eight months, and my job searches had turned up empty. It felt a little irresponsible climbing a mountain instead of finding a job but I wasn't making much progress and needed a bit of a break. It would be something interesting to talk about at interviews upon my return. I had to console myself with the idea that hiking mountains to raise money for charity and to raise my own spirits was my work for this week. Instead I brought a journal, an eight-by-eight-inch book full of lined paper with "You can cover great distances one step at a time" on the cover. It was full of lists, which often included "get a job."

Unemployment didn't suit me. I had been working since I was eleven, babysitting around the neighborhood to be able to pay for little things I wanted. By age fourteen, I had a steady gig in a bagel shop, bringing home garbage bags full of the round carb bombs to help feed our family. My shoes smelled of rotten cream cheese that had dropped on them while I was smearing it on other people's sandwiches.

Middle school is tough for any kid—tougher still for one who is overweight. To put it mildly, I was definitely not in the cool club. Instead, I was taunted by older, more popular girls, who found me to be a big, easy target, too obvious to miss. They wrote fake love letters from boys they suspected I liked—"I can't stop thinking of your chunky belly. Let's go out."—and passed them to me in the lunchroom. For a moment, I would think they were real. But when I saw the gaggle of girls smirking across the room, I shrunk inside.

I always thought people would get nicer after middle school, but it seemed that each year brought a new rejection or humiliation. In high school, I never had a boyfriend, and I never went to the prom. Instead, I had a job bagging groceries at the local supermarket.

It wasn't until after college that I started to find my professional footing. Journalism drew me in because writing was my only true strength. It came easily and it seemed interesting. I was a big girl—at twenty-two, I crossed the three-hundred-pound mark. I felt like I really needed to prove myself since I was so heavy. There are so many stereotypes of how fat workers are lazy or unproductive. I was neither. I landed a newspaper gig covering crime. At the very least, it finally gave me interesting stories to tell at cocktail parties. Being a journalist with a pen pushed behind my ear made me feel confident, like the cool girl I never was. People wanted to know me.

A decade later, when our newsroom staff was cut in half and I found myself unemployed, I started to feel more and more like the awkward teen I used to be, uninteresting and unliked. Despite being married, I also felt economically vulnerable. Will I have to take my daughter out of the preschool she loves? What if that check bounces? What if my husband loses his job, too? What if we lose our home?

I didn't want to trouble my husband with these worries, or let on that I was lying awake at night recalculating account balances in my head. He had enough on his plate working full-time to support us. We mostly kept our finances separate anyway, and I hated having to ask for money for costs I would normally cover: new tires for our car, a haircut for our daughter.

With all this worry, I had trouble staying positive. I'd always been a self-help book junkie. I especially liked the ones with "If you believe, you will achieve" mantras. After being downsized, I couldn't stand that hocus-pocus. I couldn't even go to yoga, and not because I was the heaviest one in the class. The thought of hearing the words "Believe to achieve" made me want to hurl, especially in Downward-Facing Dog.

I was a good person, I'd paid my dues, but that didn't seem to matter. As much as I wanted to, it was getting tougher to believe in karma.

I badly needed an escape. Luckily, given my jobless state, Global

Alliance for Africa covered the cost of my trip because of the $20,000 I had raised for AIDS orphans in the past. Also, my three hiking companions and I were poised to bring in an additional $25,000 on this trip, enough money to build a library. I hoped the good I was putting into the world would translate to a little good karma for me.

I hoped just going up the mountain could possibly help me figure out my next steps. I found myself chanting, "I'm doing this for charity," when telling people about the trip. The first time I hiked the mountain, one of the benefits of taking a charity climb was that it deflected all the questions about how I was dropping pounds. This time, I hoped it distracted people from the fact that I was still fat.

There was something about taking on a cause such as this and announcing it to the world. It was a way of crying out, "Please, I'm good. Please see me as something other than the three-hundred-pound blob that I am. Please know I'm worthy. I am kind. I am motivated. I'm not the lazy stereotype you picture when you see someone encased in a mountain of fat." The charity climb was, in part, a way to give myself a gold star—a way of feeling better.

OUR FIRST VENTURE WAS TO a giraffe-feeding farm, which was essentially a two-story porch, where we could hold out food for them to snatch. Their tongues were black slugs, their eyes were friendly and kind.

We took videos of Tracey and Stacey holding the food in their mouth. The giraffe came in and swooped it out, as they giggled. "You're making out with a giraffe," I said.

As we were leaving, I went down to the ground level to share one last handful with one that had bent over. I couldn't help but notice their bloated bellies. I had never seen fat giraffes. Their fur was stretched over like a too tight giraffe-print sweat suit.

"Do you think they've had enough?" I asked the woman selling the food.

"They're just pregnant," she said, shrugging her shoulders.

After picking up some postcards, I looked back at the giraffes before loading into the van. I didn't think they were pregnant. They were just fat.

THE REAL REASON WE STARTED our journey in Nairobi was to visit the Kibera slum to meet female entrepreneurs, who were making a living because of the Alliance's microfinance grants, and the library the Global Alliance for Africa had built there.

In the midst of the jagged metal shacks and open sewers of Kibera, there it stood: a place of hope. While the money we raised for this hike also funded other programs, we could see, in a very tangible way, what $30,000 could do to make people's lives better. The library upstairs was lined with books and desks. Every seat was taken. On the ground floor, there was a community room. During our visit, parents were learning about HIV/AIDS, including methods for talking to their children about the disease. The meeting started and ended with song, which echoed out of the room and into the rows of shacks that these people called home.

There was also a place for female crafters to work: a corner of the library, no bigger than one bay of children's bookshelves at my hometown Summit Free Public Library. These women earned their living making jewelry and scarves to sell in more affluent sections of the city. The rest of the floor was devoted to desks for earnest students, who were all bent over books. For some of the residents, this was the only building with books that they had ever seen in their lives. I stood watching, feeling proud that I had contributed to something that would forever change them.

After seeing the library, we visited a woman running a fruit stand funded by Global Alliance for Africa's microfinancing program.

A loan of $200, which she had already repaid, got her started and now she had enough income to feed her family and take in orphans as well. She invited us to her home, and we followed her down crooked alleyways and jagged paths to a gate that creaked when it opened. Five people were living in a space no bigger than my living room. Where do they all sleep? I wondered. She showed us the benches that were their beds. Each one had a different sheet covering it, which was almost transparent when it moved.

As we walked down the alleyways back to the van, we were surrounded by girls, including one named Oprah and another named Hope.

"Here you go," I said, handing out Silly Bandz bracelets, the kind my daughter loved to give and receive in school. One dropped to the ground. "Oops," I said, picking it back up. Touching their hands, the same size as Anna's, made me long for her. I just wanted to be with her. I imagined what she was doing, playing out at my in-laws' farm in Indiana where she and my husband were staying, blowing bubbles, making ice cream, and twisting her Silly Bandz around her wrist. I felt compelled to hug the little girls, hoping it would feel like holding Anna. I missed her so much it was as if someone had scooped out my heart.

Tracey played with the schoolgirls, showing them a clapping game where they went around tapping each other's hands, trying to keep up with the speed of the game. If you didn't clap the next person's hand in time, you lost. I joined in and just loved it, being lost in this moment of play, of being present with these kids. Tracey was often like the gym teacher who made you do the extra pull-up, or the mile run. The thing you didn't necessarily want to do. But you still liked her afterward because she showed you that you could do it. She was great at getting people to participate. Even the girls who shied away at first eventually joined in.

As we walked through the slum, I wondered what that woman's life would be like without that fruit stand. Where would all those children live? Through our fundraising, we had the power to build a library. We had the power to make a difference. We could do anything.

As we continued walking through the muddy alleys, ducking our heads so as not to be jabbed by the shacks' sharp tin roofs, I was stepping carefully to avoid the flowing sewage on the streets below when a woman stopped me. She wore a black scarf on her head and a khaki jacket to cover her skirt, which went down to her sandals. She leaned against a knobby wooden fence and asked, "How can I be fat like you?"

I laughed nervously as she looked me up and down. I was used to that kind of comment being an insult in the United States. Men would taunt me on the sidewalks of New York City, saying, "Hey baby, I'd like a piece of that ass!"

But here, in Kenya, her question was meant as a compliment. I was at a loss and didn't know how to respond.

"All you have to do is eat too much!" I blurted, the words tumbling out of my mouth. The instant I said them, I regretted them. In famine-plagued Kenya, fat is a sign of beauty and abundance. I was filled with guilt for my overindulgence, when these people had so little.

"I want to be like you," she said, making a clicking sound with her mouth, a sign of hotness, like our catcall, and she held her arms out to show the width of my hips next to hers.

"How about you give me half and you keep half?" she said, smiling. If only it were that simple. In a perfect world, we would both get what we wanted. I would have a smaller body and she would feel abundance beyond her wildest dreams.

"Where I come from, it is too much," I said, shaking my head.

My thighs chafed as I walked back to the van. I took up two seats on the bench. I wished I thought of my fat as a blessing.

CHAPTER 10

Briefing

MARANGU, TANZANIA, KILIMANJARO MOUNTAIN
RESORT—THE NIGHT BEFORE THE THIRD CLIMB

As THE WOODEN DOOR OF Kilimanjaro Mountain Resort opened, I hoped the staff had changed since my last stay.

But as I tried to sneak in, I saw a woman look up from the front desk and notice me. Sure enough, it was the woman who helped me fix my pants.

"Ah, what a surprise. It's nice to see you again," she called from the desk. "Here to try again, huh?"

Try again. Yes. Surely the guides talk with the hotel staff. Gossip must travel up and down the mountain.

"Yes, this is the last time. I promise," I said. Blood filled my face as I blushed. I stood my ground in the hotel lobby, to have control and not succumb to the embarrassment and fear from the last climb—and the pants.

Because of my unusual size, people tend to remember me. I'm a weird thing to run into, especially on Kilimanjaro. I wanted to be anonymous without any pressure to be anything but a hiker. I wanted to blend into my surroundings, but from my experience, that isn't the way things happen when you're this big. You stand out.

We left the lobby to check out our rooms. Stacey and I shared one to cut costs, although we insisted on separate tents on the mountain for privacy.

In the room, Stacey emptied and repacked her duffle bag to make sure she had everything. She was worried about the trekking company's thirty-two-pound weight limit, so she kept taking things out and starting again.

She reminded me of a little kid before the first day of school, making sure everything was right in her backpack. She took out her comb, little plastic bags of toilet paper, and individual packets of Colgate Wisp disposable toothbrushes, and put them all back in again.

Like a game of Jenga, everything was in order and if anything was out of place, the whole bag would fall to pieces. I didn't have the heart to tell her the moment she got on the trail, the order of everything would likely fall apart no matter how hard she tried.

I checked and double-checked my things so many times before I left home that I didn't want to open my duffle bag. This time, I knew my pants fit because I had hiked in them several times before I left. If I saw Anna's cute little drawings on the plastic bags holding each day's clothing, I would probably cry. I already missed her so much.

I left Stacey and my bag, to take a minute to use the Internet in the lobby before dinner and our pre-climb briefing. It was a dial-up connection, but at least it was something. I wanted to have a few minutes online to connect with my family before becoming completely disconnected. I knew that when I stepped on the bus to the mountain the following morning, I wasn't going to be able to communicate easily with the broader world.

In the dining room, Sally was delighted to find out they had Diet Coke, something she had every day back in D.C. This was her last one for a while. She caressed it and held it up as Tracey snapped a photo. She had a bit of an addiction. But I wasn't one to judge.

Stacey, who found us in the restaurant, looked at the menu. "I wonder what they have for American food here?" she asked. She was looking for pasta, pizza, or submarine sandwiches. Instead there were curry concoctions she was sure would upset her stomach. She went for the item that was most like spaghetti.

Tracey, on the other hand, was adventurous in her travel and her palate, although at the moment she was primarily interested in carbo-loading.

This was our last meal before going on the mountain. Pasta and rice were the dominant foods on all of our plates. We did more eating than talking. I skipped drinking a Tusker, even though it's one of my favorite beers, because I had read alcohol lessens your ability to acclimate to high altitudes. Funny thing, I loved beer but could go months without it. I wished I could do the same with sweets.

After dinner, we met our climbing guides, Kenedy and Michael, in the lobby. They were the leaders of our expedition, in charge of managing a forty-porter trek, and making sure we all made it up the mountain.

When I first met Kenedy, I could see in his eyes he wasn't so sure I'd make it to the top. His gaze drifted down to my hips and then back up again. He had a nervous smile that told me he didn't want to stare. But he had to. I was too big to believe. "You've done this before?" he asked. "How did you do?"

My fellow hikers chimed in with a rallying cry of support.

"This is her third time," Sally said, as if she was proud to know me, as if she was counting on me to help her make it to the top. I felt sudden pressure mixed with fear race through me. What if I don't make it?

Kenedy gave a knowing "Mmhmm," as if he knew better than to believe her.

Michael was Kenedy's assistant, and he wasn't so sure of himself. He spent more time looking at the ground than in our eyes. He didn't say much, and I couldn't tell if he was just painfully shy or nervous about saying the wrong thing in English. His face was broad, but his eyes were soft. Kenedy was more of a Chris Rock type, a jokester. He had a muscular build, as if he had been working hard all his life. His biceps bulged out of his T-shirt. It was clear he had carried more than his fair share up the mountain.

The hotel's conference room was taken by a larger group of climbers.

So we gathered right in front of the front desk, the one place I was trying to avoid, hoping to avoid a conversation about my pants. I sat on a wicker chair, with a back curved so tight around the seat that I had to perch myself on the edge and hold my weight up in a squat-like stance. I was afraid if I pushed back, the whole thing would collapse.

In the same way that I could cite the rules of being healthy (drink lots of water, move more, and eat less), I knew how to make it up Mount Kilimanjaro: have a positive attitude, go slowly, and drink plenty of water.

So when our guides started to go over what to expect on the journey, I was haughty, stepping on what Kenedy and Michael were telling us about the mountain.

"So, be sure to pack sunscree—," Kenedy said.

"You'll want to reapply it every few hours or so. It's really high up there," I jumped in.

"Right, sunscreen," Kenedy said.

Being overconfident was one of the ways I compensated for my size, like my father who would spell out his military and academic titles just moments after meeting someone. My father showed this kind of bravado especially when he encountered people superior to him in wealth or in position. My father was born a month premature and the doctors never expected him to survive. He always was a fighter, and always will be.

When it came to my teammates, I liked being in a position of power. I liked being the one they were looking up to, since so many people looked down on me.

I had been dishing out advice to my team members for months before the trip over conference calls. I continued to do that while Kenedy was talking.

"And don't forget to add iodine to your water," I said.

"Well, we boil it," Kenedy said.

"Is a steri-pen enough?" Stacey said. She had bought one of the blue glowing sticks that was supposed to zap out bacteria at the press of a button.

"No," Kenedy and I said simultaneously.

Tracey seemed perturbed. She turned her head toward me with a look that said, "Shut up."

I knew the journey on the Rongai Route would pass the Kikelewa Cave, where we would have lunch, then go through the moorland, then the alpine desert. I knew the punishing summit attempt.

So as they started talking I zoned out. I've heard this before, I thought.

It must have shown in my body language. Sally leaned in as if she was in the middle of an interview.

Stacey's head darted back and forth to follow both Kenedy and me as we discussed the trail. She was trying to take in all the advice. Every word fed her fear of what was to come. Every word was something to worry about. I felt a twist in my stomach reminding me this was a serious journey ahead. Pay attention. I gulped down whatever last information they had despite the fact that I had not really been listening earlier.

Then came the questions about odds.

Stacey asked, "What odds do we have of making it to the top?"

"A strong heart will make it to the top," Kenedy said. "You will be all right."

FOR SOME, A KILIMANJARO HIKE is a once-in-a-lifetime experience. For me, it was something I felt I had to keep putting myself through.

It was an act of self-punishment.

It finally occurred to me that night in my hotel room that I was here at the base of the mountain again. The idea of hiking Kilimanjaro was a lot easier than the actual hiking of it.

Why was I doing this to myself again? Right, to get over my weight problem.

I was so excited I couldn't sleep. My body felt strong and ready but I was still nervous. I tossed and turned. Finally, I turned on my phone and saw that it was 1:00 AM. I figured it was too late to take an Ambien. I envied Stacey in her slumber.

I looked out at the moon and listened to the quiet murmurs of conversations in the courtyard. At least this time I wasn't stuffing myself before I faced the challenge. Though I did wonder where the lollipops were.

CHAPTER 11

Trailhead

DAY 1: NALE MORU VILLAGE, 6,397 FEET

THE RUMBLING, RAMSHACKLE BUS STOPPED with a jolt.

I'd been on it for four bumpy hours, my knees pinned to the metal seat in front of me. I stood up with a grunt worthy of an Olympic weight lifter. Except I wasn't lifting hundreds of pounds of barbells in pursuit of a medal. I was merely lifting myself from a seated position, no small feat when you weigh nearly three hundred pounds.

I stuffed my journal, full of shaky notes about how nervous I was, into my daypack along with my three liters of drinking water and packed lunch. I greeted the porters who would be helping my Kilimanjaro climbing team. We were due to set off on the remote Rongai Route (near Tanzania's border with Kenya) in an hour.

The ride had been uncomfortable, but I was dreading stepping off the bus even more than staying on it. In Tanzania, 18 percent of the population is overweight, compared to 66 percent in the United States. On Kilimanjaro, obesity is nonexistent.

As I sidestepped my way down the aisle and out the door, the bus bounced up as my foot landed on the ground with a thud. The forty-nine porters waiting outside the bus gasped as they stopped counting tents, rolling tarps, and knotting ties around equipment. I knew they weren't intending to be rude; they'd simply never seen a hiker so fat.

Wherever I went, from looking over the green pastures of Kenya in the distance to eyeing the trail ahead, forty-nine sets of eyes followed me. I walked around the Rongai trailhead area, a cluster of wooden shacks where buses or Land Cruisers with pop-up roofs bound for safari unload. I couldn't shake their stares, even as they were busy stuffing our duffle bags into protective sacks or collecting the food for our meals for six days. Many wore T-shirts with the logos of American universities or sports teams—probably gifts from previous hikers—and well-worn khaki pants. Clearly, they didn't have much, and I felt guilty that they would be carrying most of our belongings (from tents to long johns) up the mountain.

The extra weight seemed like too much for any human to bear. Then again, I was also carrying a lot myself.

I exercise almost every day. I'm used to the looks on people's faces as I turn the corner into my local YMCA and step on the elliptical machine. I can't tell if they're more concerned about my breaking the equipment or having a heart attack. I remembered my preparation for this trip to Kilimanjaro; I exercised a lot: six hours a week, twice a week, with a trainer, and I did that half marathon. I hadn't lost much weight in the process. But I did feel strong enough and ready for the mountain.

There, among the stares, I felt weak and self-conscious. It felt like their doubt was penetrating me like a laser beam. It was such a strong sensation that I tried not to move around the base camp too much. I felt out of place, like a poster child for obese Americans.

The trouble with feeling self-conscious about moving is that losing weight is a simple formula of eating less and moving more. Then again, I was never very good at math. "Thirty-minute" healthy meals, with all the chopping and prep work, end up taking a good ninety minutes, especially when I have a hungry, impatient preschooler to attend to. Know what takes thirty minutes? Domino's Pizza.

As I tried to stay out of everyone's way, I came upon a woman in one of the camp shacks, wooden structures built to support the climbers, guides, and porters. She was a bit plus-sized. She wore a yellow and orange skirt, a shirt tightly hugging her large bosom, and flip-flops as she made lunch for the porters.

Inside there were some cooking areas, but nothing more. This trailhead was far less commercial than the Marangu Gate, where there's a gift shop with everything from postcards to Kilimanjaro beer.

"You going to the summit?" she said, while cleaning out metal pots. Her daughter, about the age of my little girl, hid behind her skirt, playing peekaboo with me. I thought of Anna, staying at a farmhouse with her grandparents. I hoped I would live to see my daughter again.

"I'm going to do my best," I said.

"You are strong," she said. I wanted to feel that way. The forest ahead looked like the trails back home, with pine-like trees that blanketed the ground with burnt orange needles.

The red earth smelled rich and fertile. The air was sweet and damp. I looked up at the gray-blue sky, scanning the horizon. Kilimanjaro's peak was nowhere to be seen. We had admired it earlier from our hotel and from the road leading to the mountain, a white, snowy peak jutting through the white clouds only to disappear again, but here at the base it was behind the landscape. It takes five days' worth of trails, nearly fifty miles, to get to the top and back down again.

Sometimes when you're so close to something so big, you just can't see it.

WHEN I REJOINED MY FELLOW hikers in the gazebo, which would be the last actual wooden roof over my head for a week, I found Sally and Tracey sorting through their bags. They packed as if they were going on a race.

The two perfectly in-shape women had brought an entire satchel loaded with energy gel and bars—enough to survive on for a week. But what they couldn't prepare for was how the mountain would treat them. Despite their confidence and training, they couldn't know how they'd fare against the altitude. None of us could.

In my previous hikes, there had always been at least one person who seemed to be in great shape who had to turn back. There was no telling who it would be. All anyone could do was drink lots of water, have a positive attitude, and go slowly. The last thing can be hard for athletes who are used to trying to beat a clock. In a way, I had an advantage. I wasn't trying to win any medals. I was just trying to get to the top.

Stacey seemed a bit on edge, pulling her sleeves down over her tattooed arms. Her body was nearly covered in tattoos, like a canvas for someone else's art. She felt a little out of place, nervous about stepping outside of her home, away from where she could get anything via Amazon Prime. There would be no more shopping trips to prepare for this. She had to do with what she had.

Stacey told me that if I could take on this hike, she could, too. For her, this trip wasn't about dropping pounds. Stacey's backpack held a tiny vial of her mother's ashes, a woman who had the same gentle face and was also an intrepid traveler. Since her mother's death nine years before, Stacey had been spreading her ashes around the globe. When her father—an avid outdoorsman—was alive, Stacey had never cared to join him on his camping and fishing expeditions. She preferred to go shopping. Now that he was gone, she wanted to emulate him.

I gingerly plopped down on a bench in the far corner of the gazebo, trying to rest. I knew I needed to relax, mentally and physically, but found myself drifting into thoughts about my family. I wanted to call my husband and daughter but wasn't sure about the phone connection. I didn't want my daughter to worry if we lost each other mid-sentence.

As I scrolled through my voicemails, I noticed one from my mother, and clicked on it reluctantly. "She's totally freaking out about me going this time," I said out loud to Stacey, as I listened to my mother's trembling voice. Instead of wishing me luck, she sounded as if she was bidding me adieu on my deathbed.

"Now remember, if you feel tired, just turn back. I want you to come back." I put the phone down.

"I wish she would just wish me luck instead of doubting me." As the words left my mouth, I felt instant remorse. Here I was complaining about my mother when Stacey didn't have one. I was a complete and total asshole.

I wanted to heal my relationship with my mother before it was too late. When I was younger, I wanted her to be the mother who packed my lunches and always took care of me. But she was too distracted trying to establish a new life with a boyfriend to see me for who I was at the time. My weight gain went unchecked over the years, even though she was a nurse.

As an adult, I still didn't quite feel as if I was high on her list of priorities. She'd beg for me to visit, then pack her schedule with other events so I barely saw her when I was there.

Before the Mad Half Marathon, Chris and I invited her to join us at Bove's, one of Burlington's best Italian restaurants. She and my stepfather went to Italian Garden instead. After my parents divorced she tried to rebuild her romantic life. It was just one more time when it felt like she chose men over me.

I looked at Stacey, who looked down at her boots, which were barely broken in. She had bought Asolos, the same kind as I. They were good boots; my pair were on their third trek up the mountain.

FROM THE RONGAI TRAILHEAD, THE mountain didn't look dangerous. The base was dotted with cabins among coffee and banana plantings. If I didn't know better, I'd think we were headed for a few days of easygoing daytime walks and nighttime stays in cushy bed-and-breakfasts. But I did know better. I was worried about how Stacey would do. I even worried about Sally and Tracey, despite all their confidence.

I had brought these women here—all for the cause of raising money for Global Alliance for Africa. I was the trek leader. I felt responsible for their safety but I couldn't guarantee it. I couldn't even guarantee my own.

CHAPTER 12

Defeating Mountain

DAY 1: NALE MORU VILLAGE, 6,397 FEET—STILL

SOME SAY *KILIMANJARO* MEANS "MOUNTAIN of greatness" or "white mountain" in Swahili. *Kilma* translates directly to mountain or hill, except in the local dialect *Kileman* means "that which defeats or becomes difficult or impossible."

Either translation works. Kilimanjaro is a big, white mountain that becomes increasingly difficult to scale and could quite possibly defeat any hiker.

Like Mount St. Helens and the infamous Mount Vesuvius, which destroyed the towns of Pompeii and Herculaneum in AD 79, Kilimanjaro is a stratovolcano. Its characteristic cone shape, formed by layer upon layer of volcanic ash, hardened lava, and pumice, reaches high into the sky. When these kinds of volcanoes erupt, it is with a force like a shaken bottle of soda unleashed into the air.

The mountain is considered dormant. Its last major eruption was sometime between 150,000 and 200,000 years ago, but I figured it could blow again, possibly right when I was on top of it. Yes, that was me, spending my time worrying about what could be instead of just being. It occurred to me that was probably part of what fueled my overeating.

Anticipating all the work ahead of me, I wondered why I couldn't be the type of person who spent her vacation on a beach somewhere. Oh, yeah, because I hated being in a bathing suit.

As WE WAITED TO HEAD up the trail, I walked back and forth, making as many trips to the flushing toilet as possible, knowing it would be the last one I would see for more than a week. Each time I sat down, my pants dipped low, exposing my blue and white checked underwear. I wished I hadn't bought them on clearance. If I could have, I would have traded them in for a few pairs in khaki so they'd at least match my pants.

I felt like a fool, and I worried I looked like one, too. Not that I wasn't used to ridicule. After college, I was a target for foreigners who saw me as a big, fat green card. I had two marriage proposals by age twenty-two, from men I barely knew. Fortunately, the Scotsman was an incredible kisser. So maybe I used him a little too.

I was anxious to get going, ready to escape the eyes of the porters and other hikers and walk into the surrounding forest. Instead, we had to wait for thousands of dollars' worth of Mount Kilimanjaro National Park permits, which were tied up in a money-transfer debacle. There were several other tour company mix-ups already during the trip—a six-hour van ride (during which the van ended up getting a flat tire and involving a frightening exchange with a well-armed Kenyan police officer who didn't like Tracey taking his photo) instead of the one-hour airplane flight to the Kilimanjaro region that was in our itinerary; hotels for later in the trip were swapped out for less expensive ones—and now we were worried that our Kilimanjaro trek wasn't even going to happen.

As much as I would have loved to front the cost for the permits in order to get going, I didn't have a dime to spare on this trip. We passed the time with banter, but I, for one, was worried. Despite this, I didn't want to keep walking in front of the porters—even though I'd be walking with them for days—to ask how things were coming along.

We knew our group would be slow-moving with Stacey and me

holding us back. The first leg of our journey was supposed to be the eas-
iest, but with this delay in our start I wondered if we'd be able to reach
camp by nightfall.

Unsettled, I headed back to the gazebo, where a group of strapping
white South Africans sporting red alpine gear had taken a seat.

"Are you heading up the mountain?" one asked me. He was
silver-haired and taut-muscled. He looked like the kind of guy who
spent every weekend doing some kind of expedition—biking, hiking,
sailing—the kind of guy who would have the perfect set of matching
gear for each adventure.

"Of course," I said. I mean, why else would I have been on the
trailhead with a packed backpack, hiking boots, and poles at the ready?
It was one of those "No shit, Sherlock," moments. As when a substitute
instructor from my regular spin class would inevitably zero in on me—
and only me—and ask, "So is this your first class?"

Thinking of this filled me with frustration, and I asked the smirking hikers, with a touch of spite, "Are you?"

They turned away and whispered what I imagined were snide comments. I could hear their laughter. I knew they didn't see me as fit for
Kilimanjaro or fit in any way.

"I did walk a very hilly half marathon to prepare for this," I said
stiffly, since they seemed so convinced I wouldn't make it.

I was interrupted by our trip coordinator, who looked strangely like
Gary Coleman, handing around the ledger to sign. Crinkled and ink-
blotched from the rain and wind, the paper was scrawled with the names
of others who were already on their way up. The park service tracked each
hiker's progress. Those who make it up to Gilman's Point earn a green
certificate. Uhuru Peak, at 19,343 feet, merited a gold certificate. Both
achievements came with bragging rights.

Our goal was Gilman's Point, the roof of Africa, to watch the sun
rise over the curved horizon, then make it back down to safety. To me,
this would mean ending on top and erasing my failed second climb. I
could move beyond this mountain.

But like the promise of diet pills, could one magical trip really
change everything? I had my doubts, but it didn't matter. At this point,

with my bags packed and my hiking boots on, it was too late to turn back. Our group of four signed in, knowing that most likely, at least one of us would not make it to the top. I guessed everyone thought that person would be me.

As we milled around, the porters passed out boxed lunches. The plastic bins were tightly packed with food. They weighed a few pounds. Michael took them out of the bag and plunked them in our hands. We were supposed to eat them halfway through our initial four-hour trek to our first campsite, but because of our permit delay we'd have to eat now.

I hated eating in front of people I didn't know.

In general, my binges were done with such speed and secrecy that nearly everyone, even my trainer, would say, "But you eat healthy. I've seen what you eat."

But really, no one had seen what I really ate. I'd buy a pastry with an elaborate design of pink rose icing and put it in a paper bag. Keeping it inside the bag, I'd put my mouth on the open end and inhale the pastry in a matter of seconds. Then I'd discard the evidence—empty bags of chips and half-gallon cartons of ice cream—deep within the trash. I'd quickly buy replacements, hiding the grocery receipts deep in my purse.

I didn't want anyone to know that I, this mountain-hiking mama, could be conquered at the sight of a cupcake. Of course, it also felt a little ridiculous to pretend that I ate like everyone else on the mountain, picking at my sandwich, an orange that was actually green, and a hard-boiled egg, as the other hikers not so surreptitiously looked on.

I should have been making healthy food choices months ago. Perhaps then, the wooden board of the gazebo bench wouldn't have sagged under my girth. I used my thigh muscles to support myself and prevent a possible collapse. This was not how I should have been straining myself. The real challenges were still to come on the mountain.

Still, I almost defiantly put the egg aside. Not because I wasn't hungry, but because I wanted to prove to everyone that when it came to food, I could leave a little something behind. Then I changed my mind. This is no time to watch calories, I thought, tapping the egg. After all, over the next week, I would be walking dozens of miles, scrambling over rocks, balancing on makeshift rock bridges, pushing on for as long as fifteen hours a day. And as the air grew ever thinner, I knew that each step would become more difficult than the next.

A porter came, breathless after running up the hill from a parking spot, waving papers. They were our permits, meaning it was time to go.

I gathered up my backpack, which suddenly felt heavy, and finally settled it on my back. As I walked into the grove, twigs cracked under my heavy footsteps. I passed the warning sign at the trailhead painted in bright yellow letters. The first of a dozen or so Points to Remember read, "Hikers attempting the summit should be physically fit."

CHAPTER 13

Green Mountains

DAY 1: RONGAI ROUTE, 6,600 FEET

My first steps on the mountain were creaky. My hamstrings felt like stiff wads of day-old, already chewed bubblegum that wouldn't stretch. But bit by bit, footstep by footstep, they started to remember all the walking during my training, and loosened up for the trip.

It wasn't that walking on Kilimanjaro was easy, but because of the two hikes I'd done before, it was familiar. My calves and quadriceps worked in tandem with my legs, which resembled those of an elephant galumphing through the woods. There was both an ease and a clumsiness to moving at three hundred pounds.

I did feel a certain confidence as I watched my brown leather boots find their place on the forest floor, thudding down, sinking slightly into the mud or crunching into the orange dried pine needles. Every once in a while, I'd look up to see the blue sky breaking through the canopy several stories above me, but mostly I looked down and focused on the path in front of me.

Keeping my eyes low is something I've done since my mother moved us to Vermont when I was nine years old, where at night she worked as a nurse and during the day studied for her master's degree.

Our three-bedroom condominium, built during the early '80s construction boom in South Burlington, was at the bottom of a hill. The condos at the top of the complex had an amazing view of Lake Champlain flanked by the Adirondacks on one side, the majestic peaks of Camel's Hump, Mount Mansfield, and other Green Mountains in the other direction. From our unit, we could see the carport.

After we moved to Vermont, I lived as if something was missing or empty in my life. With my weight gain, I had crossed into the Pretty Plus section of Sears, and I never came back.

From my very first day in my new Vermont school, I tried so hard to fit in with other fourth graders that when the long line of girls was finished at the monkey bars, I thought I'd give it a try. I had been a superstar at climbing on a metal horizontal ladder in Canada. But during my time in New York, as I weathered the uncertainty of my parents' life together, I stopped climbing. I stopped doing much of anything, except hiding in the pantry eating, listening in on my parents' fights, yet trying not to hear.

When I grasped the cold metal bar, my body sank down with my extra, unexpected weight. I had gained at least twenty pounds within the eighteen months since leaving Canada. My body hung like an anvil. My muscles gave way.

Focusing on holding fast to the cold metal bar above my head, it was as if I'd forgotten how to slide my feet back to safety. I was dangling, flailing, my grip slowly growing slack, my body growing sweaty. I wanted to scream "Help!" hoping someone would catch me, but I also didn't want to draw attention to myself.

I breathed like a panicked dog as my fingers slipped and I hit the ground with a thud that knocked the wind out of me. My head clunked on the cement pad holding the bars in place. I was out cold.

I didn't want to see the entire school circled around me, whispering and giggling, wondering if the new girl was alive. Then I felt the teacher on recess duty touch my arm. I couldn't look her or anyone in the eye.

"Let's get you up," she said. I didn't say anything. I just walked with her, arm in arm, to the nurse's office.

I stayed there, stretched out on a cot, staring at the ceiling, until my mother came to pick me up before her evening shift. When I saw her, I wanted to explain what had happened but it all came out as breathy sobs.

"I tried," sob, "and then," breath, "I fell."

She took me home. I rested with an icepack on my lumpy head until I had to go back to school the next day. From then on, I was someone who didn't quite fit in. And it only got worse.

Three years later, I crawled like a Marine from in front of the couch, where I had been watching MTV lying on my belly on the floor. The front door creaked open and thudded against the wall of our entryway. As sneakers squeaked against the linoleum floor, I tried to figure out who had just arrived.

I was spending my twelfth birthday watching music videos, something I did frequently because I lived vicariously through them. I wanted to step into A-Ha's "Take on Me" video. I would swoon over Madonna's "Crazy For You" ballad. I loved living through music so much that I was the only solo act at my school's lip-sync contest, mouthing Irene Cara's "What a Feeling" song from *Flashdance*.

But on this day, I was grounded for trying to host a party in the woods the weekend before my birthday. My mother told me not to have the party, thinking there was something fishy about it, but I did it anyway.

My friend Berta told everyone in school to tell me they would join me in the woods to celebrate my birthday. That night, when she and I walked into the woods, I was filled with excitement. I was looking forward to a night with friends. I even brought a pitcher of Kool-Aid and a bag of potato chips. But it was all a big joke. No one was coming. I stood there alone with Berta, who came up with the whole evil plan just to hurt my feelings. She unveiled that it was all a big joke, cackling like a witch, scaring away the birds singing their evening songs. I was crushed. Then my mother, who heard from a neighbor I was going ahead with the gathering, came up the path. I was grounded for not listening to her and heeding her warning.

Back at home, I was face-to-face with an intruder's dark, hairy legs. It wasn't until I looked up that I saw it was my oldest brother's friend Darren.

When I saw him, I felt like the air had been knocked out of me—not in a good way. He once threw me against the wall in his home when I was trying to protect his younger sister from being pummeled. I can still feel my shoulder denting the drywall, my head jerking back with a thud before landing on the mustard shag carpet. He ripped at his sister's hair and railed on her with fists of fury. Each time I saw his face after that, I heard her scream, and felt myself being thrown into the wall again.

Then, my mind drifted to the time Darren snapped my other brother Derek's nose. Derek had made the mistake of throwing a snowball at him, a typical consequence of playing outdoors in Vermont in the winter, but Darren leapt on him like a cougar. I can still remember the blood dripping on the snow as Derek ran inside to safety. I stood there frozen, too afraid to scream or move, fearing I would be next.

And yet, Bryan thought he was cool, fun to be around. Both he and Darren strove to be the sort of delinquent that you would find in the movie *The Breakfast Club*. Both Bryan and Darren were finding their way through life with absent fathers, but Darren was a friend that I wished he would drop. Bryan was a lovable puppy dog at his core, seeking attention and affection from whomever he could get it, to a fault.

I imagined Darren would one day run a pit bull fighting ring, torture people for ransom, or live surrounded by the four walls of a cell block. But today, on my twelfth birthday, he was climbing over the couch to get to me.

He saw me, on the floor facing the TV and sat on the couch, directly over me. His legs trapped mine, like a small cage.

Then he started to rub his foot up and down my leg. Slowly at first, so I thought it was a mistake, as if his foot had just fallen there. Then his strokes became more deliberate, his toes inched under my shorts and into my crotch.

Before I could say anything, he landed next to me, pinned my hip down with one hand, and held my face with the other. His mouth covered mine. His tongue fished in and out, like a koi thrashing about on dry land.

His hand moved down to my shorts and dove deep into my panties. He pawed and poked.

What was he doing? I wondered. None of it was remotely fun. I couldn't breathe. My nose was reluctant to take in his horrible teenage body odor, and his mouth (with unbrushed teeth) was completely over mine. In the beginning, I didn't fight him off. I just wondered what on earth he was doing. I couldn't figure it out.

My sexual experience had only gone as far as crushes on the celebrities in *Teen Beat* magazine. I had the hots for Michael J. Fox in *Back to the Future* and Tom Cruise. I'd made out with my pillow a few times but that's as far as it went.

I hadn't even had my period yet. I was just a kid, so it was all very weird to be watching MTV and have someone climb on top of me, pawing down my pants, sticking his tongue in my mouth. I didn't scream. I mean, he was my brother's friend. Surely, he would stop or my brother would stop him.

A few minutes into it, Bryan walked in and saw us. Then he walked upstairs.

Save me, I thought. Save me!

My brother was wrapped up in his own teenage vices, such as sneaking vodka from our parents' liquor cabinets and trying whatever drugs came his way. In truth, I think he was afraid of Darren, too. When Darren was in a rage, he would throw records like Chinese throwing stars. I became more and more anxious after my brother went upstairs. I couldn't yell for help because Darren's mouth consumed mine. I was stiff as a board as he pawed down my panties and into my flesh. Slowly, I checked out. This couldn't be real.

Like Dorothy clicking her heels, I kept thinking, I shouldn't be here. I shouldn't be here. It was a mantra I said again and again in my mind. I shouldn't be here.

So when he leaned up to unbuckle his ripped-knee jeans, I found a moment to get out. I quickly freed my knees, rolled out of his pouncing reach, and hopped up onto my feet. I bolted to the kitchen as if nothing had happened and wiped my mouth with my forearm to get the taste of his tongue out of it.

I opened the door of the pantry; its squeak was deafening. I pulled out saltines and peanut butter.

"Do you want something?" I said.

"I'm good," he replied, as he huffed upstairs, unable to finish what he started. Food had saved me.

He cornered me two other times that week, and again I cut it short by bolting up to go to the bathroom or the kitchen. One night, worried he would be back, I lugged my dresser across the carpet of my room to block my bedroom door. I watched the minutes tick closer and closer to 11:31 PM, the time my mother typically returned from the evening shift.

I wasn't even sure if Darren was in our home, but I moved my dresser, opened my door, and ran into my mother's room, next to mine. I dove under her blankets and pulled myself close to her as if I was once again a toddler afraid of thunderstorms.

She asked, "What's wrong, honey?"

I didn't know how to explain it.

"I'm sorry, Mommy," I said. "I'm so sorry."

I told her what happened. I knew it was wrong. I just didn't know why. It felt awful, and I was scared I would get in trouble. Like this was my fault.

"I'm sorry too. Stay here," she said. She dialed zero on the rotary phone by her bed and got instructions from the police dispatcher about how to file a report. I found my place in her bed, nestled below the blankets.

The next morning, we went to the police department.

I sat in a room with a friendly officer, tall, handsome, and strong, the same guy I had seen give talks around our school about stranger danger and bike helmets. I had to show him on a drawing, an outline of a body, where Darren had touched me.

I sat there shivering, even though it was mid-June, as my mother and the officer went in the corner and talked. We decided to press charges, and Darren went away to reform school for a while. As soon as he came back, Bryan went back to hanging out with him, but had to do so at his house.

Darren only came back to our home one other time. It was for a meeting with our mothers in our living room to clear the air. Mom, who had suggested the meeting to get closure, lit candles. It was her nature as a psychiatric nurse to talk things through—to process.

I dug deep into the cheese plate she had put out. I let the Ritz crackers melt in my mouth so I didn't drown out the conversation with their crunch. It sounded like a sonic pulse going on inside me.

I don't remember much about the conversation except that Darren downplayed his actions by talking about images he had seen in magazines. His mother apologized. Darren blamed society.

"Sex is everywhere," he said. I wanted to hide my head in my shoulders.

I always wondered why my brother had not come to my rescue. Later Bryan told me he thought we were just hooking up, apparently something Darren did often while Bryan was around, so he didn't want to disturb him. To this day, I fantasize about my brother ripping him off of me and drowning him in the stream behind our condo, being my hero. I feel like there is still a chance for the whole scenario to have changed—to have been stopped.

Darren never touched me again. I came home and kept the lights off, squirreled away with my snacks, which I would tuck on a ledge between my bed and the white walls of my bedroom. I'd crunch on the snacks incessantly while watching music videos.

I gained forty pounds that summer. By August I broke out with shingles, a chicken pox–related ailment typically reserved for senior citizens or those who have depressed immune systems.

Those red, hot sores were like buzzers to my nervous system, rising up to jolt me every time I sat down or when my shirt rubbed them the wrong way. I remember seeing them in the mirror, trailing down my back in a jagged diagonal line, like the shingles of a house.

The next year at school I walked around most of the time with my head slumped down. Shame was a shroud that I carried with me always. It was heavy, and I made myself heavier by dipping into every available snack bowl and bag of chips. My appetite was voracious.

Darren's sister and her friends, including the fake party planner Berta, made matters much worse by telling kids in school that I went to the police. Darren's sister sided with her brother, of course. Some of the mean boys in school, especially Joe, a kid with a major Napoleon complex, and Chad, who I later learned had his own demons at home, led all the teasing in school like a pack of hyenas and used this knowledge as ammo. They ate alive any kid who showed the slightest insecurity. I was one of their favorites.

They thought the fact that I was abused was funny, and every time they saw me (out of earshot of a teacher) they chanted, "Sexual harassment, stop, drop, and roll."

They found me in dark corridors lined with lockers. I was terrified to be seen outside of a classroom. When I saw Joe and Chad, I tried to make myself invisible, because I just didn't want to hear their torments. The punishing, ridiculously stupid refrain bore right into me. It was as if I was being punished for telling, for doing the right thing. I feared even going to school and had more than a dozen absences because I just didn't want to be there. I couldn't be there. But unfortunately I had to be.

It was especially bad on my thirteenth birthday. The anniversary of what had happened. In wood shop, the entire class giggled as Joe and Chad went on again.

"Sexual harassment, stop, drop, and roll." This time they added a new favorite, miming an erection when I was around and saying, "Bing, Kaaaara."

I couldn't breathe, and I ran out of the classroom unexcused to go to the principal's office. I couldn't be there anymore. My mother picked me up before heading to work.

I went home and perused the cleaning products, trying to figure out what would be the most lethal—to see which one I wanted to end it all.

CHAPTER 14

Bearing

DAY 1: RONGAI ROUTE, 6,900 FEET

There is a big difference between planning a trip and actually being on it. The packing, the immunizations, and the training all lead up to this journey, but once you're on the trail, there is no turning back.

I fielded Sally's, Tracey's, and Stacey's questions for months about what to pack and what to wear. On this first day, we all wore zip-off hiking pants, as I instructed, ready to spring into capri mode if the weather turned hot and steamy.

We were starting out all clean and dry with neatly folded clothing in our packs. Our bodies were clean and shaved where they needed to be. Our fingernails were pristine. But from here on out, I knew they would be like dirt mops, collecting every little bit of dust that we passed.

We were in the thick of the rain forest, each step taking us further and further away from creature comforts. We were purposefully moving away from the hassles and troubles it took to get there, moving away from our jobs—or lack of jobs—higher up the mountain. We were at a place where everyone was equal.

I came to new realizations with each passing moment. Realizations like it's one thing to test out gear in a store, but it's very different to be actually wearing it on the mountain. There was no going back to the resort for a wardrobe change or to REI for one final bit of outdoor protection.

Our zip-off pants were the only thing between us and the elements. In fact, the steady swishing of our pant legs was the only real sound out on the quiet trail other than the thud of our boots on the ground. We were going at a wedding march pace, almost in unison, along an unassuming trail that was relatively flat. It was a good way to ease into the difficulties to come.

Sally was nice, sweet, professional in the real world, but today she was like a schoolgirl. She had waited years to take on this challenge, and she wanted to get going. Finally, in the year of her fiftieth birthday, she was doing it. Although, funnily enough, she never did say she was turning fifty. It was mostly referred to as the "five-oh" or the "big milestone," but never just the number.

"I wasn't prepared for it to be this slow," Sally said. She wasn't complaining; Sally was too polite for that. It was that kind of poise that got her through interviews with the president of the United States. She covered disasters such as Hurricane Katrina in New Orleans, where she grew up, with grace and calm. She was raised a southern belle, but on the inside she was a badass warrior, an athlete. She had trained hard, and she marched like a soldier, doing whatever Kenedy said to do to get up the mountain. Her diligence and grit had gotten her through some impressive athletic challenges.

Tracey was a by-the-book athlete. If there was a challenge in front of her, she read about it, worked with the pros (from trainers to teams), and conquered it. With a mix of scientific approach and old-fashioned grit, she would get it done.

"I'll walk slow if he wants. I'll walk backward if he wants. I'll do whatever he says to get up this mountain," Tracey said.

Tracey sported a heart-rate monitor and carried a Garmin, which tracked the altitude and other mountain conditions. She was an event planner by trade. Everything she did was planned, calculated, and orchestrated. Her gadgets were her guardian angels. She even relied on their numbers to plan her snacks—energy gel or Rice Krispie treats—and this hike was no different. There was one thing she couldn't control, however, and that was the altitude.

I interrupted her downward Garmin gazing by saying, "Look for monkeys in the trees."

Tracey immediately perked up. "There's a monkey in the tree?!"

"Well, somewhere," I said, hoping to find one to point out, although all I could see was the green canopy of the forest that was starting to envelop us. "Yeah, you should see a monkey eventually."

"If you don't see today, maybe you will see one on the last day," Kenedy said. The last day—a full week away, seemed like an eternity. Each day was dependent upon the next.

But first we had to get used to where we were.

We were all urban creatures. Sally and Tracey lived in Washington, D.C.; Stacey was from Boston; and I was from the suburbs of New York City. Just being outdoors was a treat, but it also felt foreign. There were no train schedules, no traffic lights. There was just the power of our own feet.

Tracey looked up. "Did you hear the roosters this morning?"

"I did. Good wake-up call," I said, as a couple of hikers from another group blasted past us.

Immediately, I thought to myself, Gosh, they are really way more fit than I am. Then I thought, Suckers, you're not going to make it because you're going too fast.

I tried to combat those vindictive thoughts with positive ones. Eventually, I settled on "The slower you go, the better." But we couldn't go too slowly. There was a schedule to stay on.

Tracey—ever the training machine—had set her watch alarm to go off every fifteen minutes to remind her to drink.

At first, it sounded like a college drinking game, all of us calling down the line, "Drink!" as the mechanical beeping disturbed our conversations and pierced the silence. But after the first six times, it was annoying. Couldn't she remember to drink on her own? Wasn't an alarm set to go off every fifteen minutes overkill?

I was about to spend six nonstop days with these people. What if I couldn't stand them?

My mind drifted to math. Every fifteen minutes added up to four times an hour with as many as twelve hours of hiking in a day for six days. My nose scrunched up as I looked upward, as if the answer was in the trees above me. I reached in my pocket, thinking about pulling out my iPhone to use the calculator. Instead, I continued to work it out in my head. I can do this. Four times twelve is forty-eight. Forty-eight times six is almost three hundred.

I wanted to tell her to stop, but this was something that she held on to, a technique to get her through the climb. I was going to have to relax.

Beep. Beep. Beep.

"Drink," Tracey said. "Hey, Kenedy, is there any kind of poison ivy or poison plant I should be on the lookout for?"

Up at the front of the line, Kenedy had an expression on his face that made it clear he didn't understand the question. "Huh?"

"Are there poisonous plants?" Sally asked. "That make your skin itch, or give you a rash."

"Yes, Michael has it," Kenedy said, referring to his assistant guide, who was making sure no one fell behind.

"No, no, no. They're wondering if there is a plant, something that is bad," I clarified.

"Something that will make you scratch," Tracey said.

"Here on this route, no. They west of Kilimanjaro," Kenedy said.

At that time a crew of porters passed us with our stuff on their heads. Even with the gear weighing them down, they could move much faster than us, being stronger and acclimated to the altitude. I could see my duffle bag and felt immediately guilty that I wasn't carrying it myself.

"Let the porters pass. Always give them the right-of-way," I said, turning back. Sally and Tracey applauded their effort.

"Yay," Sally said, and then she mustered up some of the few Swahili words she knew.

"*Asante sana*," she said. It meant "Thank you."

"*Asante sana*," I echoed. And I felt it. I couldn't be on this mountain without them. "I love the porters."

I did love the porters, but I also felt uncomfortable around them. I thought about the way they looked at me with a "What is she doing here?" gaze. That look made me feel unworthy of this trip, ashamed of what I had made of myself. I was a glutton. The fact that I couldn't understand their language fueled my insecurities.

I remembered something a yoga teacher once told me, "Stay out of your mind. It's a bad neighborhood."

She was right. But I would be spending this whole trip in my mind, working through my issues. If there was a break in conversation, I let my mind shift into a mantra: "I believe" with one step. "In me" with the next.

I thought back to my training routine: the spinning classes, the half marathon, the yoga, and the strength training, reminding myself that I was ready to be there, even if people weren't ready to see me.

CHAPTER 15

Facing Truth

SOUTH BURLINGTON, VT, 1992

Two hours into the hike and sweat was already beading along and running down my wide forehead. I wished I had worn shorts in this rain forest section of the trail. The greens all around and the moisture, which allowed crops to grow, made it feel like the inside of a terrarium.

I crinkled my nose and reached up to drag my bandana down my face, then push it back up to hold my hair, hoping no one would notice. As my hands, already dirty from the bus ride and gripping my hiking poles, felt the contours of my face, I was reminded once again how much it was like my father's.

Every time I looked in the mirror, I saw him. His broad forehead. His gray-blue eyes. His square chin and almost cowlick across his forehead. I was my father's daughter.

I didn't know this because he'd visit when I was a kid, but because he gave me a photo of himself. The polished dark wood framed his professional portrait in his master's degree graduation robes from Queen's University.

I put it on top of the pine play hutch that he gave me for Christmas the same year as the arm-long candy canes. I figured the photo would let anyone who visited my room know immediately that I had a father, even if they didn't see him in my home. I would talk about my dad as the war hero that he was. He was in the Special Forces, and he survived being shot and stabbed several times. I was proud of him. I was proud that he was half of me.

But months would go by without a phone call or visit, which made me think he wasn't so proud of me. Every time the phone rang, I prayed it was him. I'd put the beige receiver to my ear with a smile on my face, and the life would drip out of me when I heard a professional voice ask for my mother.

When he did call there wasn't much to say—especially when he and my mother reminded me how expensive long distance calls were.

"Ask your father where my check is," my mother would half whisper, desperation in her eyes. I would see her scribbling notes on her desk, something that looked like a subtraction problem that always went down to zero. Only now do I realize it was her check ledger.

I was her last resort to get what she needed, sent in like a bomb robot because surely my father would explode upon hearing such a question from me.

Still, I'd wrap the coiled phone cord around my finger trying to find the words to ask for the check. There were none. I couldn't ask. I was afraid the thin phone cord was the only connection between us, and I just didn't know what to say. I didn't want to anger him. We didn't live in the same house, so he could decide one day to never call again. This radio silence was all we had. Even though I wanted my father to call, I had a hard time talking to him. Part of the trouble was trying to figure out what he wanted to hear. So much happened in the weeks between each phone call—from getting teased on the way home by a gaggle of girls on banana-seat bikes to sneaking money out of my mother's purse for snacks—it was hard to know where to begin. I pressed my head against the kitchen wall. I considered telling him whom I had a crush on, but that wasn't very adult conversation.

In his absence, I found myself fixated on male teachers, especially

Mr. Swanson. I wanted to do well. I wanted to be the teacher's pet. I would look for ways to help out, even clearing the blackboard after class.

Mr. Swanson was a science teacher and tall, with broad shoulders. He had sandy brown hair and looked a bit like I imagined my father did as a young man. Mr. Swanson took a break from working as a police officer to work in the schools. I loved his sense of authority in class.

I thrust my hand up in the air anytime I had an inkling of an answer to a question, just so he would talk to me.

I was lonely in my house. I missed my father. There was something inherently broken about our family—in an otherwise intact suburban town. I had no one for daddy-daughter dances. I had no one to police my homework and check that I was doing it right, especially because my mother worked at night.

My dad really could have helped. He was a math genius. He'd open books with formulas that lasted for pages. He had shelves of these books in his home. He was always working on one advanced degree or another.

Instead, his homework help was sending me books beyond my years. He sent me a signed Gloria Steinem book at age thirteen.

"To Kara, In Sisterhood, Gloria Steinem."

The fact that he had time to visit Gloria Steinem at a book signing and not me made me feel like I wasn't on top of his list. I wish he'd call just to check in and follow up on my day. I had bad days when I felt like I didn't fit in and wished I had someone there in the evening to help me sort it out. Instead, I had to simmer with it until I fell asleep, which was when my mother returned from work. I second-guessed every gesture, suspected everything, even when he had the best intentions.

He also sent me things that I'd already outgrown, like a Care Bear three years after I was into them.

I wished he'd take notice of anything. Like the smell of smoke on my brother's Members Only jacket that I borrowed when I went to the woods to try a cigarette. Or the way I used my babysitting money to buy extravagant gifts for popular kids. Not that my mother didn't do her best, but I needed a father, a gatekeeper. I needed someone to say, "You can't go out dressed like that."

Not that dressing too scantily was a problem in any case. After I was molested, I only went out in turtlenecks and covered every part of me I could. He knew I had been sexually assaulted but did nothing other than threaten to kill Darren once over the phone. I just wanted to be held.

Despite my awkwardness, I found ways of making myself feel successful. I worked a part-time job, was a bench warmer on the varsity soccer team and even earned the Coaches Award for coming to every game with a positive attitude, and I started the Amnesty International chapter for my school. I volunteered everywhere and any way I could. I even got decent grades. Except in math.

By high school, I even had a nice group of friends: Bridget, also from a broken home; Julia, a Swedish tennis star who was living in town while her father worked at the local university; Heather, an adventurous artist; and Megan, a smart hardworking girl who was Irish through and through (and honor-society studious). There was also Christie, a doe-eyed girl whom the boys liked, but she was just a little too quirky to fit in with the Benetton crowd. After graduating middle school, I had also graduated to shopping at Lane Bryant, an adult plus-size store.

When my dad did show up for big events in my life, he seemed to have a way of making them difficult. On high school graduation day, I had the alphabetic good fortune of being seated next to my best friends Bridget and Julia. I had always wondered if that was the reason we'd become so close in the first place. Our last names started with "R," so we were always seated next to each other in class.

I scratched my head, itchy from my fresh perm, and adjusted the bobby pins keeping my powder-blue graduation cap in place.

"My dad is here," I said, craning my neck to find him in the crowd. Of course, Julia and Bridget knew this. I had been talking up his visit for weeks. On this unusually steamy day in June, I was excited to know my father was here. Even if it was with my stepmother Helen, a woman who yelled at us for walking too close to the furniture and made us a week's worth of food using cream of chicken soup recipes, in tow.

Still, he'd made it. I wanted to sit in a way that would make him feel proud. No slouching. I adjusted my back on the folding chair. I pulled the graduation gown down away from my neck so it wouldn't choke me and straightened my spine. I was six feet tall—the tallest girl in my class—and I hoped he could see each little adjustment of my body by the top of my graduation cap.

We sat through an address from our co-valedictorians—Dawn and Lauren—two best friends who loved learning. They said something about living life to the max, which seemed odd since I only ever saw them studying in school.

Then, we sat through the class awards. I wasn't selected for any. I was a solid B-average student, naturally smart, but left to my own devices at home, I didn't put in a lot of effort. Writing came easily to me, with my grandmother on my father's side, who moved to Vermont to be closer to us, being an aspiring novelist, nudging and encouraging that skill.

On the other hand, I was lucky to pass Algebra, mostly because I gave up on doing the homework. I longed for a father to put the fear of God in me if I didn't have my homework done by the time he got home, someone who would tell me that there would be hell to pay. Hell to pay.

Just once I wish someone had said, "Just wait till your father comes home."

I tried to be an advanced student. I even signed up for AP Chemistry because I had done so well in biology. My first test score was an F—smack on the top of the pile for everyone to see. Quietly, I dropped the class and never mentioned it to either parent.

With neither parent paying particular attention to me academically, I was left to push myself. I was at the mercy of my own awful inner voice, a voice that harangued me with warnings of how people would react if they knew I lived in a little condo in this rich town, or that I had been working since age twelve, or worse, that I ate whenever I had a quiet moment. Just keep trudging on, I told myself. That's what I did.

During graduation, even as I walked across the stage to get my diploma, I worried that my dad wouldn't be proud of me. How could he be? He didn't really know me.

Stop that, I thought to myself. He's here. Of course he's proud. I'm his daughter. I'm graduating.

Then the superintendent called my name, "Kara Lynn Richardson."

It was a name given to me by my two parents. I wondered if it took them a long time to decide or if it was something they came up with on the spur of the moment of my birth, when they met me. I'd never thought to ask.

On this day, my name was announced on a loudspeaker so everyone could hear—even two people sitting on opposite sides of the gymnasium. They could both be proud of that name. That girl. That high school graduate.

I was whole, at least for the moment of walking across the stage, knowing that I was off to great things. I returned to my seat glowing, with a diploma case in hand. My fingers proudly rubbed over the silver finish of the royal blue frame of the document.

Afterward, we poured out of the gymnasium, trying to find our parents. My friends and I stuck together and ended up on the front lawn of South Burlington High School. The school's tile exterior looked like a '70s bathroom renovation gone bad.

As we gathered and parents found us, it seemed like a natural spot to pose for photos. My mother took a few with her windup camera.

Each one of us had a pink carnation and a fern. We all stood, clutching our diplomas. I looked for my father in the crowd. I hoped I'd spy him taking photos. Carload after carload of families left the school, and I was still there waiting for him.

I had seen my father in the crowd, but he disappeared. I was still looking around when my friends finally dispersed. My mother sucked in the side of her lips. I could see a wave of disappointment move through her. I tried to ignore it as I smiled and looked at the waning crowd around me. I figured it was just because she didn't really want to see my father.

My new black Naturalizer flats my mother bought me for the occasion grew damp from standing in the grass. The Band-Aid on the back of my heel got soggy and made the blister below it sore.

My mother, standing near me, coaxed me along. "Come on, honey. We have to meet people at home."

Of course, that's where my father was, I thought. He must have gone straight to my house to celebrate with us. He always wanted a jump on traffic. He hated traffic. He always yelled at it when I was a little kid.

So we piled into our beige Honda Civic, which was rusted around the wheels. I held my carnation and fern on my lap, treating them with delicacy as if I was holding the Miss Universe bouquet. As my mother pulled into the condominium parking lot, I scanned the parking spaces for my father's car. It wasn't there. I looked back to see if he had parked on the street. Still nothing.

He must have gotten lost. He's not familiar with the area, I thought.

As angry as I had been at my father over the years, the thought of seeing him made me giddy. My daddy. I felt the same way that my daughter does when she waits at the window for Chris to come home. I was excited and hoped to feel the love that I grew up with, but also terrified I would end up feeling the same void I had the past several years.

My mother turned on the light above the pine table that became hers in the divorce agreement. The pine dining table, the one I had to sneak by when I was molested, the one that marked his absence each dinnertime when there were just four family members instead of five. Over the years, she had turned the condo into a home, with a woodsy cottage feeling with high-end crafts for decoration. The light made the grocery store cake's icing glisten. Pretty roses along the sides looked ready to sprout out of the confection.

For once, I could wait to eat. My brothers and grandmother made chitchat, while I looked out the kitchen window. I noticed every rustle of grass, hoping it was my father's car. The parking lot was so full of cars, it was difficult to see, but none was his.

I didn't want to cut the cake until my dad arrived. He was a special guest. And with all the emotional negotiating I had to do to make this a joint event instead of two separate graduation parties, I didn't want to start without him, even if my stepmother would be there too.

My brothers didn't want to look me in the eyes. They knew. He hadn't been in their lives either. Bryan's art and mechanical expertise and Derek's stellar academic performance had gone unnoticed. It was as if they were deleted from my father's to-do list.

After about an hour, he still wasn't there. So I called his hotel room.

"Don, uh, Dr. Don Richardson, please," I said to the front desk attendant. I hoped he wouldn't pick up.

"Yes," he answered, as if at the helm of a ship.

"Where are you?" I asked, looking out the window, still hoping I'd see his car pull in, even as I heard his words at the end of the line.

"We're not coming," he said gruffly as if I was supposed to already know that.

"What do you mean?" I said.

"We left because you didn't get any of the awards," he said. "We came all this way and you didn't get any honors. Quite frankly, I'm embarrassed."

"What?" I said, my voice shaking. "I just graduated."

I wanted to throw up. Instead, I threw the phone down, nearly pulling the contraption from the wall. Merely graduating wasn't good enough.

My mother could see my disappointment. My heart thumped with rage. I kept my eyes fixed on the carpet. I knew if my eyes met my mother's, I would burst into tears, and I had suffered enough humiliation that day.

"Let's cut the cake," I said, and handed my mother the knife.

I took the knife from her and sliced through the layers of icing and vanilla cake as that phone call had sliced through my heart. My bottom lip quivered. I tried to hold it together while everyone was looking at me.

My mother gave me her "I'm sorry you're disappointed again" look, her head tilted to the side and a pout scrunching her lips.

"It's okay. I'm okay," I said.

"His loss," she said, as I grabbed for the biggest slice of cake. Suddenly, I couldn't get to it fast enough. I finished it like a bear bent over a pile of Snickers at a campsite.

I used my finger to mop up any crumbs from the paper plate. Then, as I went to talk with my grandmother, I pulled my finger across the cake's cardboard base to pick up any frosting left from the other pieces and stuck it in my mouth.

I went upstairs and sat on my bed, an antique that my mother and father had picked out when I was a child. The wood was engraved with swirls, and the coils below the mattress squeaked as I sank down. I picked up the photo of my father in a master's degree graduation robe on my hutch, and I hurled it across the room. Wood bits from the frame flew everywhere.

CHAPTER 16

Sweet Fix

DAY 1: RONGAI ROUTE, 6,900 FEET—TWO HOURS IN

WE CAME UPON A FARMHOUSE on the trail with a few rows of vegetables
to the side poking up emerald green through the dusty soil. The wooden
structure looked wobbly, with holes in the wallboards. Our English chat-
ter and the crunch of our hiking poles attracted the attention of three
kids, who came running toward us. Their hands outstretched, they called
out perhaps the only word they knew in English, "Chocolate."

One boy, no older than eight years old, was wearing a tattered man's
T-shirt that was so long I couldn't tell if there were pants underneath.
The middle child, a girl probably about four, wore a filthy purple sweater
with holes in the shoulders and a pink hat. The youngest was wearing
pajamas, which for her seemed to be all-day clothes, and a green hat that
fastened around her neck. It looked as if they had been wearing the same
clothes for weeks.

The kids had learned most hikers carried chocolate with them
in their packed lunches, tiny Cadbury bars that aren't really necessary
energy-wise to eat on the first day with the fairly light six-mile hike to
the first camp.

I just couldn't get away from sweets, even on the trail.

"Do you think it is okay if I give them some of these candies?" asked Sally, with a handful of butterscotch disks in her hand.

"Maybe we should give them lollipops," I said, pulling them out of my backpack's side pocket. I wanted to get rid of them as soon as possible, so they wouldn't be with me for every snack break, or alone with me in the tent in the dark nights.

"Here, let me get it ready for you," I said to the little boy, taking off the wrapper. He put his hand out, as if asking for another.

I gave a lollipop to the littlest girl. She was so young it was likely she had just learned to walk. Sally handed a butterscotch candy to the older girl.

"That's it. That's all I've got. I only brought a little bit. I wish I had more for you," I said, relieved to be rid of the sweets.

Sally, who doesn't have children but adores her nieces, took one last candy out for the youngest. "Here's one more. I'll put it in your pocket."

She tapped the pocket, though it looked as if the candy would wobble out.

"*Asante,*" the elder girl whispered. While I watched the children run to their shack, I realized that the coloring books and crayons I had intended to give them were sitting in my stowed luggage at the bottom of the mountain. Somehow, the lollipops had made it in the bag. The crayons would have been brighter and lasted so much longer.

I zipped up the empty side pocket of my backpack after double-checking that it was indeed empty, a sort of OCD survey of sweets. Then we all stepped together, past the farm and into the trees, passing around a travel-size bottle of sanitizer to clean our hands.

I wondered what my hiking companions thought about that exchange. I wondered if they noticed, or if they thought less of me for having brought candy in the first place.

Everyone else gave the kids candy, so why was it wrong for me to? I imagined they were thinking the candy was for me. It was another bad choice people could judge me for.

It's the same kind of problem I ran into at home, when I'm not sure if I messed up by eating a snack. Was it protein? Was it under two hundred calories? Have I completely messed up my day? What were the guides thinking?

I felt the same way I do on Halloween back home. I hate trick-or-treating with my daughter. I worry that parents will think it's really all for me. Sometimes I even make bold sweeping announcements at the grocery store, "No, honey, that has too much sugar," so everyone in the cereal aisle will think I'm making a good decision for once.

The thing about having an eating problem is that you have to eat no matter what. It's not like being an alcoholic or a smoker, where you can quit cold turkey. Food is a necessity. How much food, though, is another question.

In the forest, we saw colobus monkeys hopping from branch to branch and a stream trickling in the distance. I wanted to listen to myself even if my thoughts were not what I wanted to hear.

This was a rare thing for me, to be alone with my thoughts, my body. Normally, I was constantly noshing to get away from both.

The hours of constant grazing, little snacks I tell myself won't add up to much: a handful of cereal here, a yogurt there. But they do. I'm full but I'm still empty.

If I wasn't chewing on food, then I'd chew sugarless gum to numb my thoughts. Or else I'd drink coffee or water, which drove me to the bathroom every fifteen or twenty minutes.

I spent all my time stuffing. Stuffing. Stuffing.

When I was fourteen, my mother found Swiss Colony catalogues and candy wrappers stashed beneath my bed, like a teenager's stash of porn. I had tried to get a credit account with Swiss Colony to order the towers of petit fours and bonbons.

"Kara," my mother said, shaking her head with a frustrated sigh, when the credit department called to say my application was declined because I was a minor.

On weekends, I'd walk to the Freidhoffer's Bakery outlet near my middle school. They had great prices there—ten treats for one dollar. I'd load my backpack with cream horns and lemon iced pie pockets. I told myself I'd only eat two or five. Instead, I ate until I felt like I couldn't take in any more, and then I ate some more. I stuffed the wrappers deep in my closet to hide the evidence.

Sometimes I wanted to erase what I'd done. Change the past. Make it better. But I couldn't erase the shame. I could never hide from myself. I could never hide what I was doing to myself from the scale.

Even with all my hiding, I wasn't fooling anyone. I never was. With each year, more pounds would pile on. Despite all my secrecy, my eating never has and never will be a secret.

I wanted everyone to believe that I was okay because I didn't believe I was worth the time it might take for someone to take care of me. I'm just fine. I got this. If I'm not fine, then people wouldn't want to bother with me, to work with me, to be my friend, or family.

On the mountain, I was free from the endless routine of emptying bags and replacing them again. There were no convenience stores. No candy drawers. No secret stashes.

Here, food was just food, just energy. Had I not brought the lollipops, these six days of hiking ahead would be very, very relaxing. Instead, they became one more thing for me to beat myself up about.

As I THOUGHT ABOUT ALL this, my walking slowed, as if my difficult thoughts were holding me back.

"Everything okay, Mama Kubwa?" Kenedy asked. He looked at his watch, recognizing it was late in the afternoon. Even though this was supposed to be an easygoing first day of hiking, we needed to motor along.

We were only a few hours into our trek, and I could see he was already worried about me, as he looked me up and down again.

"Want me to carry your backpack?" he said.

I wanted to just be one of the hikers. I just needed to walk. Every time Kenedy offered me special help and made suggestions, knowing that I had already been up this same exact path, it reminded me that I was huge.

CHAPTER 17

Love Letter

DAY 1: LATE AFTERNOON, RONGAI ROUTE, 7,500 FEET

FINALLY, WE REACHED THE LUNCH site. There were two picnic tables along the trail. Most people arrive there by lunchtime so it's a nice place to stop. However, we were there much later. I sat down on the picnic bench next to a babbling brook. Sally and Tracey shared a different bench. Stacey found a spot to adjust her overflowing daypack. As we sat, we were like Lilliputians surrounded by bushes that could easily swallow us.

Another group of porters paraded by. Taking the opportunity to play getting-to-know-you, our head guide Kenedy asked, "Are you married?"

"Yes, to a wonderful man named Chris. He's back home with our daughter," I said. I always felt like people were a bit incredulous whenever I told them I was married. Kenedy's lips twitched sideways in a fake smile, as if he didn't believe me.

"Actually, it's good you're leading us up the mountain. I'm terrible with directions and I'm lost without him," I said.

Kenedy's reaction made me doubt my own words. As if it couldn't be possible someone could love a fat person. But I was loved, regardless of the fact that twenty years after I was molested, I continued to put myself in danger by carrying all this weight. By trying to protect myself in a way that wasn't protection at all.

I was en route to making Chris a widower, never mind leaving Anna motherless. In a way, it made sense. I never thought I deserved my husband's love. I kept waiting for the other boot to drop as if our marriage was a ruse, a game to trick me, like the frat boys in college who would hook up with me as a dare.

I weighed more than two hundred pounds by the end of high school and topped out at more than three hundred pounds in college. Over the ensuing years, I gained and lost as many as one hundred twenty pounds, my mounds and ripples of cellulite compounded by birthing a child.

For me, food became not just protection against unwanted advances of men but comfort, solace in good times and bad. It was also my torturer. With each pound I gained I loved myself less.

If anyone expressed appreciation for my form, not that it happened often, I'd shrug off the kind words and the rare compliments. Even when the compliments were truly well-meaning, they were often of the "You have such a beautiful face" variety. (Translation: "You'd be a whole lot prettier if you lost weight.")

Once, working out at my local community center, all 360 pounds of me chugging along on the stationary bike, I was approached by an elderly man. I saw him there each week; he spent more time talking with people than he did exercising, but he seemed lovely and harmless. As he got closer, I could see the number tattooed on his arm, marking him as a Holocaust survivor. I never asked him about it directly, but I knew what it was.

"Where I come from in Poland, you would be the most beautiful girl in town," he said, as I sweated and huffed. He went on to explain that the big girls were a sign of abundance and wealth, something that was scarce in his time.

I blushed on top of my exercise flush, and not because I was flattered.

I was humiliated. I tried to use fat to hide, but instead, it seemed to make people feel free to say whatever they were thinking.

However much I weighed, I never felt safe and secure with my body around men. With any advance, even a minor one like a stranger calling me "honey" or "sweetie," I get mad. My hands clench and my shoulders rise. If someone lurches in for a European-style greeting kiss, I freeze and sometimes land right on his or her mouth by accident.

Most comments about my body were intended either as an insult or a joke. Most people get to escape the torments of middle school once they outgrow it. For heavy people, they continue—for life.

I'd hear, "Nice ass!" while walking down the street in my neighborhood, then turn around to see a saucy teenager, surrounded by his guffawing friends, pointing at my posterior.

I hated being big, but I didn't know how to stop this cycle of feeding my emotions. Being fat was who I was. The ironic thing was, I had someone at home who really loved me and not because he had a fetish for fat girls.

Chris's love always surprised and delighted me. When I met him, I weighed solidly above the three-hundred-pound mark. I was dating his best friend Drew, who spent a lot of time watching *X-Files* and *Simpsons* reruns. We slept together after twenty-five-cent draft night at a college bar. I had pockets full of quarters. We just kept dating after that.

I was comfortably numb in the relationship, and on food. Drew would order enough Chinese food for a family of eight. And then we'd go to town on cold sesame noodles and barbecued spare ribs. Drew flunked out of the University of Vermont twice. I loved him because he loved me back.

Chris would periodically walk up into Drew's attic room in his mother's house. He was a breath of fresh air in the smoky attic. Eventually, Drew broke up with me, saying, "You're so big because you have such a big heart."

Fuck off, I thought.

Still, I found myself trying to play footsie with him at times, working my way back into his bed for a romp when he felt like it. I was a freelance friend with benefits but I often found myself heartbroken. I thought I wouldn't meet anyone else and that eventually Drew would change his mind.

Chris and I saw Drew was going down a bad road. He would wake up at 2:00 PM to go work at a restaurant and party the rest of the night. Apparently, his family was also concerned. His father sent him away to Hong Kong to work with a mentor to learn the world of finance. He didn't stay in finance long. Instead, he found a wife, an authoritative Austrian who eventually convinced him to cut his hair and straighten out his ways.

When Drew left, Chris and I had each other. I liked him in a dear friend way, in a way that I would tell him everything. I was the one person other than his mother he would confide the little things in. Like "I have a rash under my arm. Should I get it checked out?"

It wasn't a romantic relationship, but it was intimate. I brought a red gerbera daisy to his doorstep the day that the Knicks lost the playoffs—not realizing that it was the same day his cat died. He almost started crying at the sight of the flower, saying, "How did you know?"

AFTER DREW LEFT, OUR TIME together became much more active. Of course, at times we would eat too much Chinese food and keep up with must-see TV—all the way from the beginning of *Friends* to the last moment of *ER*—but I even exercised with Chris, walking while he ran. It felt very healthy. I loved coming to the end of the path and having someone there to meet me.

I went through a few relationships, if you could call them that. There was the roadie from California who would ask me to call him every night for phone sex, tell me he loved me, and then didn't want to be seen out in public with me when I visited him in Santa Barbara.

When Chris started dating someone named Elizabeth, who was twenty years older than he was, I started to feel jealous. She had money and could afford to take him on vacations where he could pursue his Middlebury literary dreams as a writer. But when she pushed for commitment, he fled.

"It just wouldn't work out," he said, as we ate at Boston Market. I smiled a little and pushed some sweet potatoes in my mouth, looking down at my new sneakers. My other ones had worn out after so many walks in his neighborhood.

I was drawn to Chris; I had to admit it. I felt giddy when he called. My heart pounded when he came in the room, but I was afraid to push it. I didn't want to ruin this amazing thing that had come into my life. I was starting to feel healthy. I felt like there was someone invested in my well-being.

I hated being in my own place, even though it was only the next town over, without him. I didn't want to be back in my latchkey world. He was my family, friend, and confidant all in one. When I broke my foot while walking the child I nannied home, he was the one who took me to the hospital—and then to Häagen-Dazs after.

I had no one to shower with affection so I spent my energy on Chris.

We were meeting our friend Jenn at Chili's. Chris was late, so it was just Jenn and I sitting at the bar at first. She wasn't known for hiding her feelings, and said, "Isn't it about time you two got together?"

I was thinking the same thing. But instead of saying anything, I took another sip of my margarita.

It wasn't until the night of my college graduation, right before I was about to move across country to take my first job as a newspaper reporter in Ventura, California, that things started moving in a romantic direction.

My friends and I decided to celebrate my graduation with a party at the house where I was a live-in nanny. The parents and kids left for the evening, so we didn't have to worry about ending the party early. My friend Bridget knew I liked Chris and picked up a bottle of Popov Vodka to help move things along. When things wound down, we retreated to my room, as if it was what we always did.

We settled into bed as if we'd done it a million times, the tension and bliss of talking with our faces so close. I don't even remember what we were talking about. We were just filling the time with nervous words before the inevitable hookup. I was nervous and excited. It was all rushing by me like a speeding car, but finally I mustered up my courage and looked in his eyes. Eventually, I said, "What if I kissed you right now?"

It was bold, perhaps vodka-fueled, but it was what I really wanted. And so I did.

There was nothing scary about being intimate with Chris. To

be side by side with his body for the evening felt natural and safe—especially because he didn't push me to have sex. After we stopped kissing, I slept softly in the cusp of his arm.

Then I woke up and worried that I had ruined everything. I scurried out of my room and down the hall to find Bridget, spilling the details as Chris slept in my bed.

And even though it was 9:00 AM, and most of us were still nursing hangovers, Chris picked up the microphone from the karaoke machine we rented for the graduation party.

The living room was filled with the Cars' "Drive".

The soft '80s beat, synthesizer, and Chris's voice trying to mimic Benjamin Orr crashed into my heart and filled me up. I turned, and I nearly cried.

Holy crap, this thing is for real. It's really happening, I thought. His voice scratched through the cheap speaker system:

> Who's gonna pick you up
> When you fall
> Who's gonna hang it up
> When you call
> Who's gonna pay attention
> To your dreams

I was in a dream. I couldn't believe this was happening to me, to the fat girl who got turned down by every guy at every dance. Maybe he just liked the song. Maybe it wasn't for me.

But when it finished, with the warm glow of the synthesizer, Chris smiled at me.

Thank God he didn't regret it, I thought.

I didn't either.

Still, I was afraid to jump up and hug him, fearing he didn't want anyone to know what had happened.

We never looked back from that day on. I did go off to California for a new job, and we had a long distance relationship for a while. He sent me mix tapes, with songs relating to some kind of thoughtful theme: my journey to California or the death of my grandmother.

On Valentine's Day, a mix tape came with a baggie of red foil-covered Dove hearts. I melted. I would play the music he sent to me over and over again in my room. I wanted to be surrounded by him.

Sometimes, we'd have virtual movie dates. He'd watch the late show on the East Coast, and I'd watch the early show on the West Coast. Then we'd call each other so we'd have something in common to talk about.

He came to visit me, including right before New Year's to ring in the year 2000, when many were worried the world would end or there would be a big Y2K computer problem. We went to Universal Studios anyway to celebrate, and the world didn't end.

I wanted to be back on the East Coast, so after a year, I applied for jobs at newspapers in New Jersey and landed a gig at *The Star-Ledger* (a coup for a relatively new reporter) and they offered to fly me back home. I took so many trips back to New Jersey that the guy at the Continental gate recognized me on that last trip between Los Angeles and Newark.

EVEN AFTER ALL OUR YEARS together—fifteen years now—I still can't quite accept Chris's love. I can't believe it's true. I've never been able to believe that my husband loves my ripples and curves. At best, I've always assumed he loves me in spite of my body, and I'm constantly on alert for signs that he is ashamed of me, that he seeks to put distance between us when I come into a room.

But he never does. None of it is true. It's just in my head.

When it came to weight loss, I wanted so much to please my husband. It was heartbreaking for both of us when I couldn't make progress. It wasn't anything he asked or begged for. I just thought, to be a good wife, I should be slender—more arm candy than sneaking candy. At the gym, I took classes with trophy wife types, who sweated their way through spinning just as I did. The only difference, I reckoned, was that between classes I fortified myself with candy binges instead of raw juice regimens. Given how difficult it felt to lift each leg on the mountain, I wished I'd downed more raw juices.

I had a loving family, yet I still thought of myself, of my body, as a big fat joke.

Again and again, Chris and his family have filled a void in my life. They are stable and loving.

My husband is nothing like my father, who'd hit on waitresses right in front of me. He'd give some floozy more attention than he gave me, while I ordered dessert. After six years of marriage, I worried that Chris's love would just vanish. After all, who could truly love a morbidly obese woman? Even when he blows me air kisses and lingers in bed to snuggle, I can't help wondering, is this real? I fret he's already gone.

Each little nag felt like a wedge between us, as if I announced I was not lovable and he should seek elsewhere for love.

When he talks about someone at work, a female, I worry he secretly wants his life with her, not me. When he had a short stint using chewing tobacco, I imagined him dying of tongue cancer.

We pledged to be together for life, but I worry that he's only in it for the short term. That's not based on anything he has said, but on my own fears.

It would be wonderful if the act of his coming home, of just showing up every day, could be enough to convince me that our relationship is for real. We have a child together.

Not feeling worthy of my father's love made me fear the loss of my husband's. It was as if somewhere in my heart, I felt our marriage was doomed before it began. That was my path. But my husband is not my father. He is good for me. Despite my size, we fit together.

Back on the mountain, I closed my eyes for a moment and believed I was attractive. I believed I was loved fully, as was my round yet strong, supple body.

And yes, I was married to a wonderful man named Chris.

CHAPTER 18

Bucket List

DAY 1: MOORLAND CAMP, 8,530 FEET—SUNDOWN

WHILE THE DARKNESS SETTLED ON that first day on the trail, the flickers of light from the campground ahead grew brighter. But they weren't bright enough to illuminate the ground in front of us.

We weren't supposed to be out on the trail in the fading light. Otherwise, we wouldn't have left our flashlights in our backpacks. On a dark trail, there is no way to see the ridges and roots below. You have to trust the next step won't send you tumbling into a volcanic stream, or you won't twist your ankle on a rock.

"So much for night vision," Tracey mumbled, as it became harder and harder to see. She said her legs felt strong, her knees were okay, but a headache was brewing, certainly a result of the noticeably thinner air.

She told us about her friend Laurel, who had hiked the mountain a few years before being diagnosed with Parkinson's disease. Now, her friend had trouble getting the groceries. When things got tough, Tracey vowed, she would focus on Laurel. It was her prayer, her meditation.

"Mmm," I acknowledged, trying to focus on Kenedy's footsteps in front of me. Our trail chat grew quiet as everyone tried to concentrate. The first day out was supposed to be casual, fun. Instead, it was turning treacherous in the growing darkness.

I listened to the slow sound of my boots thudding on the rocks, willing myself not to fall. If I went down, all three hundred pounds of me, I worried that my bones would snap on impact. With each step I wobbled, bracing myself with my poles. The horizon disappeared into the darkness. All that remained were the crescent moon and a blanket of stars.

Despite taking this path twice before, I couldn't remember it. There was so much to this mountain that each curve was still a surprise. I only remembered it in snapshots, like a highlight reel in my mind, but I knew that there was a lot of lost footage to cover in the days ahead.

As we drew closer, the porters heard our soft curses, calls of "Oh, shit" and "Fuck!" each time one of us almost took a dive. They came out to greet us where the path met the campsite, a relatively flat swath of land. They held up their own headlamps to light the way.

"Better late than never," I said, scanning for my tent. The porters had illuminated the tent strings with their flashlights; they looked like trip wires out of a James Bond movie. Sometimes you saw them, sometimes you didn't. Distracted by the tent strings, I stumbled over a rock almost immediately.

"Oh, shit," I said, flinging out my arms and catching my balance just before I fell.

Normally after the first day on the trail, there is time for tea and popcorn, to go through your gear and settle into your camp. But we were so late because of the permit mix-up that we were directed straight into the mess tent for dinner. There were two groups camping at Moorland Camp that night with us: a honeymooning couple and the cocky South Africans who seemed to want nothing to do with us for the rest of the trip. Because it's less popular, the Rongai Route allowed for privacy. It's a little harder to get to because it's on the side of the mountain closest to the border of Kenya. Most people opt to hike up the Tanzania side of the mountain, but they miss out on the stellar view of Kenya from the rocky grove of this camp.

The porters set out camp seats for all the other hikers, really just a piece of cloth no bigger than a luncheon napkin held up by three plastic sticks. At my place setting, they had left a bucket, knowing I wouldn't be able to fit one cheek of my ass on the regular camp chairs. I sighed a little. But I was glad to have a place to rest.

The cook stuck a pillar candle on top of a can for light.

"This is great, having hot cocoa and tea by candlelight. This is really neat. I haven't camped in a long time. It's been like twenty-five years since I was camping with my dad. It's just nice," Stacey said, trying to take it all in.

She drew the cup up to her lip and sipped again, thinking about her dad, seemingly at peace, despite the effort it took for her not to fall over on the little camp chair. I could tell that Stacey had her doubts about whether the chair would hold her.

My bucket seemed to be holding, but I felt the need to address my strange seat with humor.

"I guess I could take this as humiliating or just be grateful," I said. "But since I'm not sitting on the ground right now, I guess I'm going to be grateful for it. I don't fit in some of the camping gear that's out there. But I'm here and made it to camp one. And I'm eating popcorn."

Tracey took a giant handful. Our hands just missed each other before I reached in again. Other than the crunching, the green mess tent was quiet. Our table was set with a tablecloth and napkins. It was a strange luxury to encounter in the outdoors. It was not exactly roughing it but not exactly glamping either.

"We are devouring it because we need the salt. It's justified," I said. "We're really hungry. I'm really hungry. I worked hard today. There are harder days to come. So I hope there's more popcorn."

I laughed to deflect attention, becoming the funny fat girl who isn't sad about the way people treat her.

Then, in the uncomfortable silence that followed, Tracey spoke.

"Actually, I think this chair is quite comfortable," she said, before taking another handful of popcorn, smiling as she chewed. I chewed my popcorn more quietly. The bucket was just one of the many uncomfortable seats in my life.

ONE OF THE MOST UNCOMFORTABLE seats I've ever sat in was in New York City two years before my final Kilimanjaro hike. I don't look like anyone's picture of a woman with an eating disorder. But there I was sitting tight—literally—my extra flab squeezing beyond a too-flimsy chair in the waiting room of the Daybreak Center's eating disorder clinic. For a moment, I worried that when my name was called, the chair would lift off the ground with me as I stood.

I thought about where I would put my hands to push up and release myself from it without overturning the side table filled with self-help pamphlets. There was no doubt that I had some kind of eating disorder.

I gazed at a girl with her mother, both of them waiting across the room in a spacious loveseat, the girl's arms barely wider than broomsticks.

It was strange for lumpy me to be lumped in with women who had the other eating disorders, the kinds that involved rejecting food. Often, the Daybreak Center waiting room consisted of me, taking up almost two chairs, plus a few sad-looking anorexic women who could have fit three to a seat. As for the normal-sized people, I figured they were bulimic.

My doctor had recommended the Daybreak Center when I broke down, head in hands, crying that I just couldn't seem to get food right. A year after my daughter's birth, I was still above the three-hundred-pound mark. My blood pressure, blood sugar, and cholesterol were normal but when it came to food, I was sick in the most shameful way, back to my habit of buying boxes of one-hundred-calorie snack packs and consuming all six in one sitting. I'd lost weight once but could not get back on track.

Every day, I sat at home, hoping my daughter would sleep, but she didn't like to nap. Instead, I would take long drives down a stretch of Route 24, praying that she'd nod off in the car. My turnaround point was a McDonald's drive-through. When she finally slept, I'd get a strawberry milkshake as my reward. By the time we got home, she'd often be awake again.

Every now and then, my therapist at Daybreak, Jacqui, filled out reports on my progress. I smiled softly, hoping my friendly demeanor would improve my report, essentially outlining Binge Eating Disorder and depression. Maybe I'm better, I hoped, but I knew that was a lie. She listened to my resentment over trying to balance motherhood and work and gave me a few coping mechanisms, suggesting Julie Morgenstern's *Time Management from the Inside Out* to help me learn to focus on work instead of using Facebook to avoid tackling my to-do list. Just that morning I'd chomped down on a softball-size muffin, even though I was full from breakfast an hour beforehand. I was already thinking about getting a smoothie on the way back home. Sometimes I told her these things. Most of the time I did not.

I craned my neck, wishing I could see the words she was writing on the fill-in-the-blank form, then looked away hoping she didn't notice my interest. I tried to be quiet; the only sound in the room was the rustling of papers.

I looked down at my computer, which was plugged into her outlet, to make sure it was charging and ready for the train ride home. Then I looked back up at Jacqui. Why was she taking so long?

Finally, she met my gaze, studying me like a listing in the Diagnostic and Statistical Manual of Mental Disorders.

"You know," she began, "the tricky thing with rating people with your eating challenges is that many of them can function just fine in most areas of their daily life. They have jobs, even high-powered ones. Like you, many have relationships. They get up and they live their lives every day. It's just that they have this thing with food," she said, touching her pen to her mouth and then putting it and her head down, almost certainly regretting thinking out loud.

I just want to be normal, to be at peace with food, I thought. I wanted to come up with some clever explanation for my behavior. We talked about my father. My abuse. They all seemed like excuses, but they were walls that separated me from how I really felt. I gulped and put my head down, studying the pattern of the tattered throw rug that had been at the feet of many clients with sad stories like mine.

I wanted my food issues to be all boxed up and put away in a neat little storage compartment, like the newly organized houses on HGTV. Instead, my issues were more like a scene from Hoarders. If you really wanted to find the root of my food issues, you had to dig through piles of mess. Frankly, I felt sorry for my therapist.

I was ten years old when my mother first signed me up for therapy, thinking it would help me cope with her divorce from my father. This was before I started gaining weight rapidly, before Darren touched me. The worst was yet to come. The therapist's name was Trina. I remember she had a set of Tarot cards wrapped in a silk scarf.

Each week, she'd encourage me to tell my fortune by laying the cards down on the floor and looking up the definitions on a tattered piece of paper.

I see now that Trina wanted to know how I'd interpret the cards to get a better idea of who I was. I tended to use them to imagine a brighter future, in the same way I loved asking questions of Magic 8 balls. I would shake it, and feel the plastic octagon clink against the plastic sphere in my hands. Finally, the liquid inside would stop sloshing to reveal answers to questions such as, "Will Diane ever be nice to me?" All I wanted was some magical message that my future would be better than my reality.

I was an outsider from Canada living in an affluent Vermont suburb. I was stuck in a condominium while the popular kids were up in giant homes on the hill with Lake Champlain views. I had to wear Pretty Plus clothes from Sears while they were in Esprit. How I wanted an Esprit sweatshirt—to wear their brand like a banner—but one sweatshirt cost as much as my mother would spend on my entire back-to-school shopping spree. I didn't fit into the clothing, anyway.

"Will I be popular this year?" I'd say to myself, holding the cards with hope, then shuffling them, dividing them into three piles, and placing them on the carpet. I wanted some source beyond me to make me thinner, richer, and more popular.

But the reality was I was the heaviest girl going into middle school, a fact that revealed itself during a very public weigh-in gym class.

I was in triple digits—120 pounds—while most of the girls weren't more than 90 pounds. I wanted to hide behind the lockers, but my granny panties were exposed. I'd get nervous changing before and after gym, my anxiety made worse by the fact that I had to take a deep breath to snap my pants closed.

The Tarot cards didn't change any of that. If I didn't get the answer I wanted, I would reshuffle the deck and start again—not that it actually helped me get a boyfriend or be thin.

Jacqui in the eating disorder clinic didn't have Tarot cards. She wasn't even supposed to have coffee—or any kind of food—in her office. She told me this when I was about to open a Diet Orange Crush. I was thirsty, so she let me have the soda. I needed the refreshment. Her office was sweltering, like an oven. Oddly, she often wore out-of-season Christmas sweaters. I wondered, but never asked, if she had food issues too. I read once that anorexics are often cold, which made sense to me since I was often hot.

I wanted to know her better. She was around my age, and had once hinted that she was ending a relationship with a boyfriend. She celebrated by taking a trip to Costa Rica with friends.

Maybe it was my reporter nature, but I kept the focus off of me by spending much of my time in therapy talking about other people. Back in grade school, I worried over my friend Cam, who was getting involved with a bad crowd in middle school. Telling Jacqui about it, I saw the real issue was how awful it felt to be losing my one and only friend. I was too heavy to fit in with Cam's new, more popular crew. When Cam was gone, I missed her freezer full of ice cream. My mother didn't always keep it in the house.

But Jacqui didn't want to hear about other people. Instead, she pushed me to get to the root of my unhappiness.

"Tell me about your father," she said.

I started to cry.

CHAPTER 19

Catered

DAY 1: MOORLAND CAMP, 8,530 FEET—SUPPERTIME

THE CHEF BROUGHT OUT CUCUMBER soup in a steaming pot. We watched as the steam danced in the candlelight, a sort of dinner show. Soup would be served each day to keep us hydrated, Kenedy told us.

This night, the entrée was fish, potatoes, and vegetables. It felt all very balanced, and I felt full eating it, but soon I was feeling a bit sick (though it was hard to tell if it was the altitude or the conversation).

"You spend time branding yourself as Fat Woman on the Mountain and then today I heard you talk about trying to cut sugar out of your life and being healthier and trying to lose weight," Tracey said.

She was referring to my website, fatwomanonthemountain.com, which I'd started a few years earlier to document my first journey up Kilimanjaro, and to help raise money for AIDS orphans. I kept it going through the second climb, when I had gained the weight back again, and again for this third, as a vehicle to raise money and tell my story.

"It seems to me that you're working this weird double angle in that you have branded your identity as fat but you're trying to continue your weight-loss efforts," she continued, her PR instincts kicking in. "What are you going to be when you lose weight and you're not fat? You will need to reimagine yourself . . . because you're not going to be Fat Woman on the Mountain, or are you?"

"So I guess I'll be Fit Woman on the Mountain," I said with a little smile, swallowing a bite of potato.

"Okay, well," Tracey said, about to continue, but I interrupted.

"That was the name of my blog because it's shocking. It's not what you expect to see out on a trail, but I suppose when I get to my goal I will be Fit Woman on the Mountain," I said.

"Don't you think it will be hard because you're living as Fat Woman on the Mountain and you're trying to make yourself fit? It's like you're psyching yourself out. You have to think about success," Tracey said.

"Well, I'm less fat than I was," I said, about to roll into how I had once topped 360 pounds, lost 120 pounds, but she already knew that. I wore that former loss like a badge of honor, but the only story I was truly living was the fact that I had gained much of that weight back.

"That's good, but," Tracey said.

I interrupted, "How about Not-Quite-as-Fat Woman on the Mountain . . . but that's kind of a long URL."

The table roared with laughter, breaking the tension between us, the uncomfortable feeling that arises when someone brings up a taboo topic.

Sally offered, "NoLongerFatWomanontheMountain.com."

Stacey chimed in with, "FormerlyKnownAsFatWomanonthe-Mountain.com."

"Then I'll become a symbol like Prince, the less-than sign," I said.

"Do you think it's going to be hard? To get out of it?" Tracey said.

"But I'm not out of it. My weight is a constant battle," I said.

"No, no, no . . . but when we do a race we are always visualizing success, visualizing coming across the finish line, just like we're all visualizing coming to the top of this mountain," Tracey said. "But when you write your blog, you're visualizing fat, you're not visualizing fit. It's a mental switch."

"Maybe I just need to sign up for FitWomanontheMountain.com," I said, with a smirk.

"If your goal is fit, that's the mindset that you need to get in now," Tracey said. "So sign up for FitWomanontheMountain.com when you get back."

"I will, when I get off the mountain," I said.

"Lock it in. Lock it in," Tracey said.

I was sick of talking about it.

"Alright, guys," Kenedy said, clapping his hands together like a coach getting his players to refocus. Michael stood back. "Alright, get some rest. Pack only sunscreen, water, and snacks in your daypack. Tomorrow will be a long day."

THE NEXT DAY WAS GOING to be a long mountain slog, as many as eight hours of hiking. As far as the weather, we needed to be ready for anything.

The only way back to our tents was via the lights of the porters. We lifted our feet over rocks and divots from campers before us, eventually finding our little yellow, nylon homes for the night, while assiduously avoiding the strings that supported them.

I chose to sleep in my own tent. I didn't want to partner up, worried I'd take up too much room. Plus, I had to pee so much from drinking as many as five liters of water each day, I didn't want to constantly wake my tentmate.

It couldn't have been later than 8:00 PM, but I didn't want to waste my flashlight or iPhone batteries to pass the time, so I shut everything down. The tent was a bit musty and smelled sweaty from previous trips, the essence of previous hikers. Now that I was in the tent, my long johns scratching at my hips, I wondered what those hikers' journeys were like. Did they sit in this nylon globe wondering if their journey would end sooner than the peak?

So many people had called this rental tent home. Now it was mine, and I needed to be comfortable with the idea that this was the best I could do for the next week.

I tossed and turned, remembering that insomnia is common at high altitude. Even when I drifted out of sleep I told myself to be still and to rest. Instead of relishing the fact that I'd gotten through the first day and felt strong, I couldn't stop thinking about what Tracey had said at dinner. Fat had been who I was for so many years.

Would people notice me or care about me if I wasn't so big? Would they notice me if I wasn't the Fat Woman on the Mountain?

I wanted to like Tracey, especially because now that we were on the mountain there was no escaping each other. But I also wanted to beat her on the mountain—her and all her gadgets—to prove that I could succeed. I turned on my iPhone to see if I had any voicemails. It kept cycling, trying to get a signal. Each minute was $5, so I quickly turned it off, sad that I couldn't just make a call to my husband and daughter to tell them that I was okay and thinking about them. But a $500 phone bill after months on unemployment wasn't a good idea.

I held the phone in my hand like a security blanket and soothed myself to sleep with self-affirmations. You can do this, Kara. You will make it up the mountain, Kara. Finally, I drifted off to sleep.

I used to sleep with my phone on my bed, next to my pillow, just in case I got a booty call. The first time I had sex was with Todd, a resident assistant at the University of Vermont, who seemed to like to break in virgins. As a college freshman, I was just the right target. Once he had me begging for his affection (I'd come to his room anytime he paged, whether it was 4:00 AM or 4:00 PM), he dropped me.

The following year, when I was a resident assistant, he started sleeping with one of the residents who lived on my floor, actually in the room next to mine. I could hear them giggling and moaning through the cinderblocks. I wished I could have turned into the Incredible Hulk and smashed through the wall. But instead, I went out sobbing in the rain to the college store and came home with Ben & Jerry's ice cream.

There's something so soothing about ice cream. If I had a favorite binge food, it would be ice cream. Sometimes digging into the cold block of cream and sugar can be challenging, but once you lift that spoon to your mouth, you almost have to smile to curve your lips around it. The cold is distracting; the cream coats your mouth.

I didn't know if they were still there when I returned from the store, but at about three o'clock in the morning I heard the door close next door. That's typically the time he called my dorm room, so I figured he was on his way to someone else.

I had a sick feeling that I was sloppy seconds to some other girl on more than one occasion. I turned over in bed but didn't sleep for the rest of the night. My fingers etched the cinderblocks again and again, a repetitive movement that I thought would strip away the mortar between them. I stared at the red digital numbers on my clock as they moved toward morning.

CHAPTER 20

Blue Baby

NIGHT 1: MOORLAND CAMP, 8,530 FEET

At midnight, with the moon high in the sky, the sound of tent zippers in the camp startled me. Then, a flashlight danced back and forth in the camp. I heard Sally's voice from the tent next to mine asking, "What's wrong?"

Tracey responded, her voice shaking, "I can't breathe. I can't breathe."

I stopped breathing once.

I was eighteen months old, although it was hard to tell below the layers of gauze covering the third-degree burns on my neck, chest, and left arm. I was in an Ottawa hospital isolation room to stave off the infections that burn patients are susceptible to and can be more dangerous than the burn itself.

Maybe it was an overdose of Demerol? Maybe it was the shock? But my little body had given up and was ready to succumb. I was alone in my hospital room, apparently stable, and my doctors and nurses had moved on to helping other patients.

My mother, who was working full-time as a cardiac nurse in the same hospital, as well as caring for my father at home after his triple bypass, happened to be on a coffee break. Haggard and exhausted, she passed clumsily through the hospital hallways from the cardiac unit to the burn center. She peeked in the window to my room, almost not wanting to look at my disfigured little body.

Immediately, she saw something was terribly wrong. I was blue. She screamed just as she did when she watched me pull the teakettle off the burner and tip it on myself.

"Help! Help! My baby isn't breathing!"

They revived me, of course. But that burn and the scars it left were the beginning of my feeling uncomfortable in my skin. My parents went to plastic surgeons in Ontario trying to find a procedure that would return my skin to its smooth, soft, peachy state. But the bubbly, thick scars on my chest, arm, and neck would always be something that made me different from everyone else.

Growing up, I had to wear a T-shirt over my bathing suit so the scar wouldn't darken in the sun, which led to a thousand questions about why I was dressed that way.

THAT NIGHT ON THE TRAIL, when I heard Tracey's pleas for help, I struggled to wiggle out of my sleeping bag, like a cat stuck in a paper sack. I couldn't get the zippers of my tent open fast enough. When I finally got all three zippers open far enough, I slid outside on my belly and hopped up to a standing position, as my trainer had me do in our workout sessions.

I shone my light on Tracey, who was gasping and pacing back and forth, trying to decide if she should go back down the mountain.

I nearly dropped my headlamp as I tried to pull it on, illuminating my frosty breath in the night air and Tracey's frantic movements. I tripped on a tent wire, then stumbled on a rock, before I got to her.

"Are you okay, are you okay?" I said in a whisper loud enough to show grave concern, quiet enough not to wake the camp. I crossed my arms over my braless chest. I was only wearing what would be comfortable in my sleeping bag. I didn't have time to find my jacket so my teeth chattered as I listened.

Even after what had happened at dinner, it was still hard for me to see Tracey, usually confident and self-assured, so frightened and vulnerable. She was like a scared puppy dog trying to explain what happened, especially when she didn't know how to explain. She spoke quickly, gasping between sentences.

"I startled myself awake and had what I can only assume was a panic attack.

"I couldn't breathe.

"I couldn't move.

"I had to get out of my tent, out of my sleeping bag, and walk around.

"I was hyperventilating.

"I was trying to figure out ways to find a trail and get down the mountain.

"It was the most terrifying moment I've ever had in my entire life," she said. "I tried to calm myself down and go back to sleep, but I guess when the oxygen level is low, and you go to sleep, you're getting even less oxygen. So each time I went to sleep, I would wake myself up thinking that I would stop breathing again."

I nodded along, trying to keep up. I wondered if I should wake up Kenedy, but I wasn't sure which tent was his. I wasn't a doctor. Neither was he. And here, it was hard to tell the difference between heightened fear and real illness.

"Did you take your Diamox?" I asked, referring to her altitude medication.

"I just did," she said, slowing down and taking a giant gulp of air. "I'm okay. I'm okay. I'm just going to go back to bed."

With that, she slipped back into her tent.

I was left standing under the stars, each one a dot over me, covering the sky.

"Um, okay," I said, as if I had played a part in her decision.

Tracey called herself a drill sergeant. She battled through excruciating physical therapy to be on the mountain. Her knee was arthritic, and doctors told her she'd never make it. This turned her into a training bulldog. I decided to trust her decision that she was okay, that she knew her body and she was in control.

Sometimes she made me uncomfortable, true, but I wanted her to succeed. Maybe it was good to have someone prodding me a little bit, questioning me. Everyone else was afraid to.

Especially me.

CHAPTER 21

Getting Up

DAY 2: MOORLAND CAMP, 8,530 FEET

THE CLANKING OF POTS AND mumbling in Swahili in the near dark outside my tent woke me up. The sunrise made the yellow nylon glow as if I was in a Japanese lantern.

I woke up lying diagonally—half on and half off the foam pad I had rented for $25. It was the only thing protecting me from the hard earth, but my body was so heavy that it pushed straight through to the roots and rocks below.

I reached for my duffle bag, tucked in the corner of my tent. I smiled when I pulled out my first plastic bag to find my daughter's stick figure drawing on the outside. I could still smell the Sharpie of my daughter's handiwork. I held the bag in my arms as if I was holding her. The fresh T-shirt—from the Mad Half Marathon—and clean underwear were plenty to smile about too. Getting dressed was like doing a horizontal mambo in the squat tent. I pulled the T-shirt over my head and lay back to tug off my long johns, replacing them with my dusty hiking pants for a second day. My socks also had to be recycled. I shook them out, instantly wishing I had done so outside, as the inside of the tent became more and more like the drum of a vacuum cleaner.

My last challenge before standing up was pulling on my boots. I groaned as I stretched down to tie the laces, my hamstrings tightening in protest as I pushed forward to loop my laces through the hooks. My fat folded at my belly, making it hard to reach my feet, but I tried to be precise with my lacing. I had at least eight hours of hiking ahead of me and any extra space in my boots could lead to blisters.

Then came the biggest challenge: getting vertical. I started with my feet in front of me, sticking out of the tent flap so I wouldn't get my tent full of more grime. Then I put one hand behind me and tried to lift myself like those Russian dancers. When that didn't work, I flipped over on my hands and knees, hoping no one was behind me as I backed out, butt first. Then I pushed up into a downward-facing dog, walking my hands up to standing, as I'd done so many times in yoga class.

I was about to utter a light "Ta-da" for any spectators who might have witnessed my ungraceful exit, but I was startled by a vision of Kilimanjaro's peak, pushing above the tree line, showing us where we were going.

It was as beautiful as I remembered, and just as daunting; it looked a day's drive away. The rambling, remote Rongai Route offered hikers more solitude and a gentler slope but it was a long slog.

I headed to the mess tent for breakfast. One by one, the dishes came out: eggs, oatmeal, toast, sausage, and fruit. There was plenty of fuel for the challenging day ahead. The team of porters took care of the cooking and cleaning up. All we would have to do was put one foot in front of the other.

As she approached the dining tent, Tracey's watch alarm went off.

"Time to drink something," she said. She was trying to flood her system with water to help with the altitude adjustment.

"I'm glad to see you're up," I said.

Kenedy was going to carry her daypack just in case. I could see her smiling, although it looked more like a wince, as she wobbled over to breakfast. She placed two hands on the table and eased herself down.

Seeing Tracey struggle made me feel guilty for feeling so strong. My legs supported my girth. I actually felt like I had energy to spare.

It was just as I'd felt four years earlier, when I was really on track with my weight. When, at 240 pounds, I felt like a success story, in control of my body and my life.

Back then, getting healthy was part of my lifestyle. Fit was who I was.

I remembered how I hopped in my car each Saturday with my Weight Watchers booklets—a weight-loss tracker, a food journal, and a nutritional information guide—all tucked in a thick black binder that was too big for my purse.

I balanced it, my wallet, and a bottle of water on my arm while getting into my burgundy Saturn sedan. Even though I had carried these with me for dozens of weeks, I resisted getting a bigger purse. I was all about getting rid of the big things in my life.

I had just tossed a batch of size twenty-eight pants in a clothing donation bin. The metal door creaked as it closed. Fitting in size twenty-four pants made me feel like a supermodel.

But I still had more to lose. My vehicle, already low to the ground, sank closer to the asphalt as I settled into my seat. My hips flowed over the center console, making it hard to plunk my drink in the cup holder or reach the CDs inside the console. Finally, I selected one from my spinning instructor: Remix Mix.

I pressed Play and my Saturn turned into a dance hall with an amped-up, clubby version of Coldplay's "Clocks" thumping. I liked high-energy music to go with the high-energy person I'd suddenly become.

With the car door closed, I could smell the sweat from my 8:00 AM workout on my skin. I spent an hour perspiring on the treadmill followed by weights—curls and lifts by the dozen. I hadn't showered before Weight Watchers. I wanted to prove that I'd been working out. Also, I was afraid I wouldn't be able to blow-dry enough of the moisture from my hair, which might add ounces to the scale during my weekly weigh-in.

As I waited for my turn at the scale, I sucked my stomach in, dipping my hand below my waistband to feel the unaccustomed space between my pants and my skin. I loved that after a decade above the three-hundred-pound mark, I was about to drop into the two hundreds.

It was all I thought about.

Whether I was commuting past New Jersey strip malls or running errands, my brain busily calculated Weight Watchers points, ounces eaten and minutes on the treadmill, hoping the coming weigh-in would see a dip in my numbers.

I was thirsty from my workout. My tongue stuck to the roof of my mouth, but I sure as hell wasn't going to have any water now. Sixteen ounces of water was a pound. So many things could work against me, and I needed to lose.

At Weight Watchers meetings, I felt like a rock star. I had to perform. Even a dip of a few ounces would draw applause and garner a sticker. I loved that gasp from the crowd when I announced how many pounds I had lost so far.

Instead of loathing me for being a fat fuck-up, my fellow dieters loved everything and anything I said. As a big loser—fifty-eight pounds in the nine months I'd been doing Weight Watchers—I was clearly winning.

The meeting leader, a forty-pound loser herself whose weight was beginning to creep back on (not that I was judging), asked, "Now, it's Memorial Day weekend. A lot of parties will be happening. What kinds of things can we do to stay on track?"

My hand shot up. "Bring a veggie tray. You can buy them at Costco all ready to go. And you can use the leftovers for veggie side dishes."

I was a teacher's pet. As if I didn't know how to add vegetables to my meals before Weight Watchers. After all, I'd read every diet book and magazine article: Eat More, Weigh Less, Lose Weight in Your Sleep. But in the past, I'd opted to let the veggies rot in my refrigerator, if I brought them home at all.

Now, when I spoke, people nodded their heads. They wanted to know my name, written proudly on a tag stuck to my shrinking chest. After the meeting, new members would circle me as if my progress would rub off on them, asking, "How long has it taken you?"

But when I stepped on the scale that week, my heart sank.

Just as I cheered my husband along on his marathons, Chris cheered me along on all my weight-loss endeavors. He was like a Boston Red Sox fan of yore, hopes rising with every season only to fall after a predictably spectacular failure.

But this time, I was making him proud.

I weighed 302, down from 360. All my pants were sagging, and I wanted a good solid number to report to my ever optimistic spouse.

This week, I didn't have it: I was up .08 pounds. All was lost, and I ate all of my One-Point Weight Watchers snacks on the way home from the failed meeting, then recorded them in my food journal. So much for my extra points for the week.

I pulled the car into Chris's parents' driveway, which led to a stately colonial home in an upper-class neighborhood. We'd been staying there while he was looking for a job. It had been almost a year, and many of the openings he pursued seemed to dry up.

I worked as a newspaper reporter, temporarily the breadwinner in our relationship. It wasn't as bad as it sounds, especially because not having to pay for food or rent allowed me to join a swank gym. Usually after I returned from my meeting, Chris and I would watch *The Biggest Loser* together. But this week, no dice.

"Didn't lose this week," I told him, my journal and wallet nestled in my arms.

"That's okay," Chris said.

And his mom helpfully added, "Maybe next week."

While some people lament their in-laws, I have to say that as a girl from a broken home, I married very well.

It took us four years to get married. I wondered if Chris was just waiting for me to get thinner before sealing the deal. But, I should have known, he's much more practical. He wanted to finish his MBA before getting hitched.

I had the husband. And even though we were living with my in-laws, it felt as if I had the home too, albeit one with a full-size bed that could barely contain the two of us. Maybe that was part of my motivation for dropping pounds. It also didn't hurt that my mother-in-law made healthy meals each night. Turkey burgers. Carrot soup. Pork tenderloin.

Sometimes, I'll admit, I felt a little bit like a misfit in this wholesome family. They were so perfect, so loving. That's why I was glad to have Chris's cousin Stacey in the mix. She lived in Boston but I saw her on holidays and family gatherings, especially after her parents died.

Like me, she was a bit broken and scarred. Her mother was in and out of mental hospitals when Stacey was a young girl. Her father—Chris's uncle—married three times before he was killed.

Stacey, fresh off a divorce, was trying to leave a boyfriend who liked playing video games more than anything else. She liked to be in control. That's why it surprised me when she signed up for the hike.

When hiking Kilimanjaro, the mountain is in control. But she reassured me that she was ready for a challenge when we took on a training week in Telluride, Colorado, in the week before the trip to Africa to acclimatize and prepare for Kilimanjaro. We even ran down Sneffels Mountain in the Rockies in the midst of a thunderstorm. We had planned to conquer Sneffels Ridge that day, but somehow we took a wrong turn on a path that led us through a mountainside loaded with wildflowers, as they often bloom with vigor in late July. We enjoyed it so much we didn't think that we were heading the wrong way.

Once we realized our mistake, we doubled back and headed up, knowing full well that late summer afternoons in the mountains meant rainstorms. As we were about to hit the clearing, the summit, the sky started to rumble. The sky was swirling clouds of gray and we couldn't remember what was safer—to be on an exposed cliff or under a tree. We figured the best thing to do was go down.

With hiking poles in hand (which we were sure would translate into lightning rods) and wobbly rocks underfoot, we started to run. The skies opened up, slicking down my shirt to each roll of my belly.

I was sweating but the constant rain rolled it all off and down my body. I wiped my brow just so I could see and keep up with Stacey. The treadmill, it seemed, had paid off for both of us.

I just tried to watch the tread of her boots so I wouldn't run into her and push her down into the mud that was quickly accumulating from the rushing water along the trail.

The forest smelled like mud and a freshly misted greenhouse. We reached the bottom safely and headed back to our condo in Mountain Lodge, happy to be in the shelter again.

"I was sure I was going to die," Stacey said to me after it was over.

LEAVING THE DINING TENT, I stuck iodine pills in my water and tried to shake up my Camelbak, which felt like a live fish as it swooshed back and forth. The brown tablets dissolved into the blue plastic water pouch.

Then Stacey said, "You do realize that we've been drinking tea without iodine all this time."

CHAPTER 22

No Trace

DAY 2: RONGAI ROUTE TO
KIKELEWA CAVES CAMP, 11,811 FEET

THE CLOUDS SOFTLY BUT SURELY erased Kilimanjaro's peak from the landscape, as they typically do on the mountain.

"It sucks that the clouds came in. I like seeing where I'm going," I said. Stacey paused in the way hikers do to emphasize a point mid-conversation, took a few more steps, and looked up.

"I think it's going to rain," Stacey said.

"I hope not," I said, sizing up the clouds in the sky. They were a soft misty gray, surrounding us on all sides, but a storm didn't seem imminent. The clouds seemed to be heading elsewhere, and the air didn't seem damp. There wasn't a dark heaviness to them as storm clouds have. "But you never know what's coming. The weather on Kilimanjaro is unpredictable."

"I have a rain jacket and rain pants. The problem is I get so hot," Stacey said. That was one of the troubles of carrying excess weight: It covers you, smothers you actually.

"Maybe it will be like a sauna. Maybe wearing it will help me drop five more pounds," I said, kind of joking but kind of hopeful.

With the view gone from the sky, it was easier to focus on the ground. The thud of our boots was like a drumbeat of progress.

The landscape was changing. We were no longer in the lush rain forest. We had entered the Moorland zone of the mountain. The plants were shorter and sparser at this point. Heather-like bushes, often no higher than our knees, lined the trail. Yellow and white wildflowers pushed through rock piles. The higher we went, the harder it was for anything to survive.

Despite the altitude, hiking with Stacey felt good. She had said my first success on the mountain inspired her, and she seemed unfazed by my second-attempt failure. It made me feel hopeful I could get back on track.

"You know when we saw that monkey back there, I was reminded that it's a good thing to be able to see things that I wouldn't have when I was more than 360 pounds," I said. Preparing for the mountain gave us a reason to be outdoors, and while I was still heavy, I didn't ever want to be back at my peak weight. It seemed 300 pounds was my tolerable limit.

"A year ago I would have sat home and watched reruns on television," Stacey said. "Now I get to be out here with the wildlife . . . and Kilimanjaro. In Telluride we got to see elk and fox. I just have a whole new appreciation for the outdoors."

Then, quietly, she started to cry.

"What's wrong?" I asked, concerned, reaching out to touch her arm.

She had started thinking about our training in Colorado. We included a road trip to Moab, Utah, to the memorial on the lonely stretch of State Route 128 where her father was stabbed to death, near the turn-off to Fisher Towers. The wooden cross held up by stones blended into the red rock background. It was a quiet reminder of a violent act, where Walter was left for dead and his assailant roared off with his truck.

It was hard for Stacey to be anywhere without thinking about it, replaying the memory in her mind, imagining his last moments. She said it was a constant and conscious effort for her to turn her thinking away from those dark places, to be present, as she had to be on Kilimanjaro.

Stacey looked out over the landscape, which was more gray than green. The vegetation, while sparser, was a delightful surprise between the rocks. It showed it could survive and thrive in adversity.

"Both my parents would have loved this," Stacey said. After her mother's death, her father watched her weight pile on.

"My dad wanted me to get out, to see and do things," Stacey said. "He was always trying to get me to go camping or biking or hiking. I think he would be glad to know that I am finally getting outside and appreciating nature. I think he would have been so proud. I think he would have thought I was crazy when I said I was going to do it."

She bent forward, crying.

"I think he's kind of been there the whole time," she said. She said she felt near him on the trail as if he was just around the next corner. "I wish I could just call them and say, 'Oh, I'm doing really well.'"

She rubbed under her sunglasses with dirty hands and got mud in her eyes. She tapped on her father's dog tag and reached toward her backpack to clutch the silver vial with her mother's ashes. She intended to take it with her all the way up the mountain.

I remembered when I learned about her father's death. My mother-in-law, Robin, Walt's sister, left a voicemail for Chris. Our answering machine was on the Berber carpet floor in our furnished basement apartment in Ann Arbor, Michigan, where Chris was in graduate school.

Robin, usually a portrait of grace and demeanor, left the message in breathy gulps, as if she was packing to rush to Utah or Ohio to be with her family, anywhere she could be helpful, while telling people the terrible news. The message was so garbled, I had to get on the floor to hear what she said.

"Chris, I have to talk with you about your uncle Walt. Something's happened. He was murdered," she said. "It was on Mother's Day."

Once I understood the words, I bolted up, leaned against the wooden entertainment center, and clutched my head. How was I going to tell Chris?

My shaking fingers botched his cell phone number three times before finally dialing his number correctly. I hoped he wasn't in class. He had a cute way of answering the phone when I called at unusual times: "What's wrong, sweetie?"

"Your uncle Walt has been murdered?" It came out like a question, as though I was wondering whether it were actually true, as though I didn't want to believe it.

"Wait, what?" he asked. "What?"

His mother and Stacey would spend the next year planning a funeral, setting trial dates, and settling the estate. The hardest thing to part with was Walt's RV, which he had used to explore the nation. But all the while on the mountain, there was grief, a constant sadness, that Walt, who would have loved to be on this adventure with us, was not there.

In a way, I felt guilty about convincing Stacey to come along, without full disclosure that she'd be faced with whatever thoughts surfaced during the hike with no easy means of escape.

We can be distracted so easily in our lives at home. We set ourselves up with food, TV, and Facebook so we don't have to face reality. Here on the mountain, Stacey had to be with herself and her memories of her parents. And so did I.

As far as my father was concerned, I wasn't quite at the point of forgiveness. In fact, thinking of my father made me walk more slowly. Why did he abandon my brothers and me when I was only nine? How did he fit into my life now?

This question always haunted me, especially in the weeks before Father's Day, when I'd stand in the greeting card aisle, looking for just the right message.

"Best Dad Ever." No.

"You're always there for me." No.

"I'm so proud to call you Dad." Maybe.

I was looking for something more like, "Thanks for forwarding me jokes every month or so."

Still, I felt compelled to buy a Father's Day card every year, hoping that our relationship could eventually rise to the Hallmark ideal, like the life I remembered before my parents' divorce.

Although he rarely sent me birthday and Christmas gifts, I always made sure to get him something. One year, I even sent him a miniature Christmas tree with tiny decorations, because I knew he would be alone.

I always made a point of sending him After Eight mints. I remembered he loved them and would let me take a few extra swanky mints, individually wrapped in a vellum envelope, when we were together. They made me feel rich.

I wanted to say to my father, "I'm thinking of you. Aren't you thinking of me?"

Most years, for my birthday, which was two days after his, he'd just call with a long-winded explanation about how broke he was.

Shortly after we moved to Vermont, when I was in fourth grade, on our only vacation with our dad, he took my two brothers and me to Washington, D.C. for Easter. The trip included Smithsonian museums, the Capitol, and the Egg Roll on the White House lawn. But what I remember most is my dad trying to wiggle out of paying for everything— from the speeding ticket he got on the way there to the Crystal Sheraton Hotel bill.

I thought about this when the porters offered to take my daypack, as they had for Stacey and Tracey. Tracey seemed to be doing better than the previous night but was less dogged in her walk up the mountain. I declined their offer. My father had let me down. Maybe that's why I didn't like to rely on anyone. Even my husband. Besides, I wasn't hurting, at least not physically. I was just slow.

Not that it wouldn't have felt great to walk around with twenty fewer pounds on my back, but I wanted to show everyone that I was fit for this challenge. I hated when people assumed that I was unable or unworthy simply because I was fat.

Stacey stopped. She wasn't feeling well.

"It's good to catch your breath," she said.

"We'll get each other through this," I said.

Two hours into the day, Stacey started throwing up repeatedly, first hunching over, then running to be sick behind a rock. She repeated the same painful routine a few minutes later.

We'd grimace as we listened to Stacey groan from a rock off trail. We offered to help, but she wanted privacy to dry heave, to be in misery.

We'd all check in with her in our own ways—trying to be concerned, but not making her focus on her ordeal. I would check in as if she was my child, with gentle inquiries like "How ya feeling?" and "Can I get you something?" Tracey was more motivational, reminding Stacey that she could do this. Sally just sympathized with a sad smile and a tilt of her head.

Michael pointed to the horizon, to the camp we were heading to off in the distance. We could make out a few tents, like pixels on a computer screen. But at least we could see the flickers of yellow.

"That's it over there—that's not too crazy," I said.

"So this isn't it for today," Stacey said after her rest. After hours of hiking and puking, she wanted to be near the end. To pack it up.

"Still something to look forward to, don't you think?"

I was trying to stay positive. I wanted to be that force for Stacey—for myself.

But already, I was starting to feel uncomfortable—as the skin chafed between my thighs. I had brought baby powder, but I had forgotten to put it on. I could feel the skin stripping away with each step, my thighs rubbing against each other and the seams of my pants. Each time I squatted to use the bathroom, my thighs burned.

Stacey and I were glad to catch up to Sally, Tracey, and Kenedy around the bend.

A cloud rolled in, making the trees look like graveyard shadows. We had been on our feet for four hours, so we found a spot on the trail where the mountain rocks formed a mini-Stonehenge. As I went to sit down on one, Michael said, "Careful, don't break it."

I laughed uncertainly as I found myself a tire-size boulder to rest my rear on.

"We like to joke," Michael said. "We've never had someone fat like you before to guide up the mountain."

"But we hope you will make it," Kenedy said.

"She's done it two times," Sally reminded them. I wanted to move on to a more comfortable subject: lunch.

"How much longer is it to the lunch spot, one hour, two hours?" Stacey asked.

"One hour," Kenedy said. He went back to his conversation with Michael—and I wondered if he, in his soft voice in Swahili, was complaining about us.

After her difficult night, I was glad to see Tracey becoming surer of herself as the day passed. She still wasn't carrying her own backpack but she was strutting ahead of Stacey and me.

I was glad she was stronger than I. She was looking as if she might have a fighting chance up this mountain after all. But then I started to think about the supplies I'd seen the porters take up. I didn't remember seeing any canisters of supplemental oxygen. When it comes to oxygen on the mountain, it's a case of Murphy's Law. You only have problems if you don't have it. I asked Kenedy about oxygen as casually as I could manage.

"We don't have any. You didn't ask for it."

"But it's standard on any trek, isn't it?"

"Not really," he said.

"We have someone in trouble. You need to get it. I don't know what it takes but that's on the tour operator," I said.

As I got agitated, I could feel my lungs tightening. I was worried, but I didn't want to waste my breath.

I had to calm down. I had to trust that our guides would take care of us. I had to trust we would get through it. There were some other climbing groups on the mountain, so if we were in distress, we could always ask for help. That is, if we didn't get too far behind. It was hard for me not to nag, not to be overly controlling. I wanted to make sure everything went according to my list, my plan. Planning and list making were the only ways I could get through being a mother, a wife, a full-time-job seeker, and a writer. I had multiple notepads of to-do lists with check boxes. Whatever didn't get done was moved to the following day, a debt of to-dos that followed me everywhere. All these to-dos made me feel important.

I felt like these hikers were in my hands. They were my tribe, people who came up the mountain because I had gotten them there. Now I worried that I'd put them in danger.

"You need to figure out a way to get some," I said to Kenedy. He immediately called his boss on a cell phone to send a runner up the mountain to meet us at the next camp. Since it wouldn't be there until the following night, I hoped Tracey would be okay. But then again we weren't so far up the mountain that she couldn't start walking back down to a lower altitude where it was easier to breathe.

Still, I worried that something could go wrong before the oxygen got to us. We were approaching 11,000 feet, and every step we took brought us closer to danger. My fellow hikers were starting to show it.

"I have these moments when I say, 'This is great, I can do this,' and then I take three steps and go 'ugh'," Tracey said.

"Glad I got the poles out," Sally said. They had borrowed some of their gear from Bob, their friend and a world traveler. There are so many things that you need for Kilimanjaro that it's best to borrow where you can.

You lean on friends to get you through the trail.

"Yeah, you got them out right at the right time," Tracey said, taking a gulp of air. She looked at the majestic, looming peak and said, "You know, Kara, you've ruined hiking for us forever. Nothing will ever compare to this."

"WE'RE ALMOST TO LUNCH," KENEDY told the group about five hours into the day.

"These are tricks they play just to keep us moving," I said. "Moving" sounded more like "move-in." I noticed my breathing was heavy from the exertion of putting down my backpack. I started dropping the last syllables of words. My hiking partners were now Trace, Stace, and Sal. This was a result of hiking higher; each step we took meant less oxygen in the air. Our lungs would crave the same rich back-home blend, but be sorely disappointed not to have the molecules to push us forward with the same strength and speed. Even the world's best athlete's performance would start to suffer under these conditions. Not that it helped me feel better about feeling so sluggish.

Stacey hunched over her poles. "I'm sorry. My stomach hurts," she said.

But Kenedy was telling the truth: after a few more steps, we could see the table set for us next to a cave. A table set in the middle of a mountain trail is a strange and wondrous thing. It was a beautiful picnic setting with soup simmering and a hot meal awaiting us. This was the only day when the chef would cook for us mid-hike. We were five hours in, and we had five more hours to go; it felt like a special occasion, a celebration of all we had done so far, which was good because I was hungry.

I tried to nudge people toward the lunch table, a little embarrassed to be focusing people on eating.

"So let's eat. I'm so hungry," I said, feeling edgy, wishing people would assemble at the lunch table so we could eat—and rest. My feet were burning. At the place set for me was the bucket. I looked for a rock instead.

Sally and Tracey checked out the rocky infrastructure of the cave, their hands smoothing over the jagged edge. Stacey tinkered with her backpack, looking for something to make her stomach feel better.

"EVERYBODY SEE THE GLACIERS? WELL, maybe it's just snow, but it's white and we're going there," I said.

"Wow," Sally said.

Wow, indeed. The glacier on top of Kilimanjaro is majestic but disappearing. It has shrunk more than 80 percent from when it was first measured in 1912. Only about a square mile of cracked ice is left and it could all be gone by 2022.

This massive hunk of ice helps the world below survive by irrigating crops and supplying drinking water to the village people. To look at it perched on the mountain is awe-inspiring, but sad. This iconic mountain, which has provided so much to so many and inspired Hemingway to write, "wide as all the world, great, high, and unbelievably white in the sun," is shrinking.

I wondered how the mountain and the people around it would survive if this massive thing weren't there. Somehow they will have to learn as it cracks, melts, and drips to oblivion.

Even things that seem as if they always have been or will be are indeed temporary. We're all moving parts, passing in and out of life. The air we breathe, the earth we stand on, and especially the people we meet are already on their way out. Still, every experience, every interaction becomes part of our DNA, our past, and our path forward.

If only I could find a way to be still, to find a way to enjoy what I had. I wanted to know that the love I had for my father was still in me. The more anger and frustration I felt for him, the more the love for him melted from my heart. The more that happened, the closer I came to losing the chance to start again, before one of us vanished.

Even Tracey, with her breathing difficulties, seemed to perk up at lunch. She settled into her camping chair and started hydrating. Her drinking alarm had just gone off.

After her breathing episode, the water alarms no longer annoyed me. They were keeping her alive.

"Drinking water makes it feel like I'm making mud in my throat because of all the dust," Tracey said.

"We have dirty hands, too," Sally said, spreading her fingers wide, showing the dirt gathering below her nails and seeping into her fingerprints.

The lunch spot was surrounded by birds picking at the food scraps left behind by other hikers, on rocks, and under the picnic table. I hoped they wouldn't swoop in and take my food. I was hungry, really hungry. It was so rare for me to feel really hungry.

The only other time I felt hungry was when I was on some kind of diet. When I ate just enough to survive, I spent my days trying to avoid seeing vending machines or any other kind of trigger that would invite me to eat. My mood was unpredictable. I often felt like I was on the edge of a cliff, leaning in, without a rope to save me.

But here, the food was just food and I ate it.

It would be five more hours locked in hiking to get to our camp for the night. An hour passed without us saying a single word. Stacey and Tracey were dug in, trying to feel better by not thinking about how crummy they felt. Sally and I knew the best way to help them was to keep on going, so we just walked.

Finally, we got to the point where camp was just over a stream and up a steep incline. The ground was mushy and soggy. The path to get us across the soggy ground was two wet, wooden planks. They had grass growing through the rainy season that was matted down by the steps of hikers. I was worried the planks wouldn't hold me.

"I don't like planks," I said in a singsong voice to hide my embarrassment. I looked downstream and saw a gigantic boulder. "Aha, an alternative route."

Kenedy traversed it first, stretching out his hand for balance. I took the boulder route too and leapt to safety over the fast-moving river. My boot came down with a thud. I often look down with embarrassment about shaking the ground below me, but that's the way I land.

"Made it. Good job, Kenedy," I said. Kenedy laughed as we turned back to hold Stacey's hand.

"Good job, too," he said.

The clouds drifted overhead. I once heard a meditation tape encouraging me to think of emotions as clouds. I didn't want the clouds to come into camp and surround us, even if they were wispy and playful. As emotions, I didn't want them to come too close. They scared me.

We truly felt like part of the sky, and the sun was about to set, casting an orange glow on the tips of the clouds.

Most times when I see a sunset, I hear my father's voice, repeating a phrase he learned in the Navy:

> *Red sky at night, sailor's delight.*
> *Red sky in the morning, sailor take warning.*

CHAPTER 23

Bet on Me

DAY 2: KIKELEWA CAVES CAMP, 11,811 FEET

At dinner, Sally, Tracey, Stacey, and I were quiet. We were tired, just waiting on the food. After ten hours on the trail, we'd run out of casual conversation.

We focused on our meal: carrot soup, spaghetti with meat sauce, and bread.

Stacey tried to eat but couldn't, still feeling the effects of her morning stomach upheaval, something that rarely happened to her at lower altitudes. Her Diamox made her fingers tingle. The altitude made her queasy.

She managed to get four bites of spaghetti down. Not being able to eat made her think of her mother going through chemo. Stacey tried to force her to eat and couldn't understand why she couldn't. Stacey helped care for her mother, who was fifty-five when cancer started in her colon and then metastasized to her liver.

As darkness crept onto the mountain, Tracey had to force herself to take deep breaths, willing calm to wash over her.

"Fingers crossed that I don't shock the camp awake and start running down the mountain the wrong way tonight," she confessed, looking down.

I was grateful but feeling guilty that I still wasn't sick. By the time I'd reached this camp during my second Kilimanjaro attempt, I was retching. Although that had a lot to do with the two pounds of chocolate I downed before leaving the hotel room.

The only thing that felt shaky was my self-esteem. I kept hearing Michael's joke from earlier that day in my head, "Don't break that rock."

I knew the guides were just trying to make light of my heaviness, but their humor was getting old. It's one thing to have made a onetime joke. But when it's a constant part of the conversation that singles me out, it starts to needle me.

Ever since bullies targeted me for telling others what Darren did to me, I always felt singled out. I worried that someone, somewhere, was making a comment against me to insult me or make me uncomfortable.

Of course, I couldn't blame the guides for making a big deal about me. A three-hundred-pound woman out on the trail is a rarity. Extraordinary, really. But I was sick of being an oddity. I was sick of exceptions, of people thinking I could crush a boulder with my girth, thinking that I couldn't keep up. I was all too aware that it wouldn't take too many more pounds before I couldn't put one foot in front of another, much less climb a mountain. No wonder people were freaking out to see me out in the wild.

I tried not to direct my anger toward Michael for his rock comment. Most times, guides just lead a group of hikers up a mountain. They don't need to worry about a hiker not having a place to sit. We headed back to our tents, stumbling over the scattered rocks. Fortunately, my tent was right next to the dining tent, so I couldn't get lost and I didn't have to walk another inch.

I brushed my teeth with toothpaste and a dry toothbrush, not wanting to waste my drinking water, and not needing to spit. I found my way to my sleeping bag in the dark, not an easy feat, and pulled on clean socks with the agility of my ninety-year-old grandmother.

The cold leaked through the tent flaps in the below-freezing weather.

We dug out duct tape. Stacey had plenty, of course, to seal up the holes. Her father would have been proud of her outdoor preparedness. We kept our cell phones close in our pockets, so they wouldn't be frozen in case of emergency. As I bundled up, my legs felt heavier than usual. The ten hours of hiking was a lot—for anyone.

I pulled on a knit sleeping hat and settled down, trying to get as comfortable as I could on the insufficient foam pad, rocks jutting through every which way. My cell phone set my tent aglow like a giant firefly. I switched it off and tried to sleep.

I sunk my hands below the waist of my underwear to hang on to my flab of belly fat. It wasn't sexual or self-deprecating. It was just warm. It was something I did most nights before bedtime. It's something to hang on to, since my hips don't let my hands fall naturally at my sides. It's also one of the few times I feel connected to my body.

I heard the voices of the porters and guides in the next tent over. They were hanging out, talking and laughing. To them, this wasn't a once-in-a-lifetime adventure; this was their twice-a-month job.

At first, the murmurs of Swahili were like white noise, since I knew only a few words, enough to exchange pleasantries. I knew that *jambo* means "hello" and *habari* means "how are you," which was often answered with a lovely *nzuri*, meaning "good."

Hakuna matata, made famous by *The Lion King*, means "No worries."

But I did understand the language of being mean. I heard Kenedy, our head guide, talking about me, "Mama Kubwa" or "Big Woman," and I knew he was laughing at me. I knew, as I listened to his grunts and groans, that he was mimicking my sounds on the trail. At first, I was mortified. I wanted to hide in my sleeping bag and not get up.

Then, I was mad. I wanted to unzip my sleeping bag and go tell him off. But what would I say? Maybe I was a laughingstock. Let them have their fun, I thought. I am an oddity. I can do this, I whispered to myself again and again until I fell asleep.

The next morning, I kept hearing that laughter in my head, those unseemly grunts and groans. Was I that ugly? Did they feel disgusted by the mere sight and sound of me? I felt humiliated and angry all over again, but we needed them to get us up and down this mountain safely.

I rolled over to my black duffle. I had placed it next to me in the night, a solid mass, pretending it was my husband Chris. Just having its familiar presence there comforted me.

Michael came to my tent door, asking if I wanted tea.

"Fine," I said.

I sat up in my tent and picked out my clothes. I'd designated my sewn-together hiking pants for the day's four-hour trek. They were clean and would do the job on the trail, but instantly I felt fat. Fatter than usual.

The memory of the guides' taunts from the night before clouded everything good in my mind. Like the fact I was at 12,000 feet, I wasn't sick, I was on a journey to raise money for AIDS orphans, and there was amazing scenery around me. The clouds moved below the mountain ridge like an ocean tide on its way to shore. The sun peeked above them, welcoming a new day on the mountain. I stood outside my tent to take it all in. To be swallowed by the beauty of Mawenzi, Kilimanjaro's sister peak, was an awesome thing. The brown, jagged peak was in stark contrast to Kilimanjaro's wide, solid top. They were sisters, but didn't look related. To know that I had gotten there on my own two feet was even better than seeing it from afar. But it didn't feel like enough in that moment.

I pulled on a little—well, not so little—black down jacket to make my way to the toilet tent and get ready for the day.

I yawned; my teeth chattered in the dry morning air. Or at least I think they did. I couldn't feel anything in my molars. Most of my teeth had been drilled down to nubs, emptied with root canals, and covered with crowns of gold and porcelain. For years, I'd blamed my dental troubles on a sealant procedure gone wrong when I was thirteen. But every new filling, under enamel that was as fragile as eggshells because of the deep decay, made it clear that the fault was my own. I had spent years bathing my teeth in sugar. Remarkably, my front teeth were still unscathed. So when I smiled, perfectly white, straight teeth shone through.

But I wasn't smiling much now. I tried to keep my mouth closed. I heard it was a way to conserve oxygen.

Standing on the mountain was like peering out the window of an airplane. Below us, Kenya looked like an agricultural quilt with patches of green and brown. Although that quilt was breathtaking, Kilimanjaro's summit in the other direction was more vivid than any postcard, any picture, any tour book. It was so huge in the background. It couldn't be denied with its stark white patches of snow and deceptively gentle but menacing slope to the ground where we stood.

It appeared more daunting, even sinister, with each step. Oddly, it felt as if we'd hiked farther away rather than closer to it.

It was like my progress—or lack thereof—on most diets. Just when I thought I had my weight under control, around the time of my first Kilimanjaro hike, I got pregnant and I let myself go. I knew all the right things to do but I just didn't do them.

I've read so many diet books that I can recite the rules of losing weight like a robot. (Which has more calories: a glazed donut or a bagel? Surprise! It's the bagel.) But instead of using my knowledge to help myself, I traveled down a self-destructive path.

When I was pregnant, I went from being someone who was capable of hiking to the top of Kilimanjaro to someone who could barely walk across my living room because of the sciatica shooting down my legs. I'd lost control of my body. And I punished myself for it. I punished myself with bacon cheeseburgers and milk shakes until I'd put on sixty pounds, half of what I'd lost, plus twenty pounds of baby weight.

Part of me wished my doctor had given me a tongue-lashing for being so fat.

However, I knew that wasn't necessarily effective. One white-haired doctor in my OB practice did give me a talking-to when I was pregnant with Anna as my weight crept back up to three hundred pounds.

"You started high. Let's not go any higher," he said. It couldn't have been more gently stated, but when he left the room, I convinced myself he didn't know anything.

I looked down at my dimpled thighs, which, given the room on the exam table, spread like blobs of marshmallow fluff.

He was full of shit. He didn't know what he was talking about. He'd never been pregnant. I thought to myself, If he's on duty when it's time to deliver, I'll just cross my big fat thighs. I fantasized about writing a letter to the practice, to the medical board even, about how wrong he was. How could he be so insensitive? But of course, he was right.

KILIMANJARO'S PEAK WAS LOOMING IN the distance, but all I could look at was my oatmeal, in a plastic camping bowl in front of me. I was perched on my bucket, trying my best to keep from falling backward.

It wasn't the yummy instant stuff I was used to. Instead of oatmeal, I thought of it as gruel, and I was lost in it, spooning it into my mouth without seeing it. I fantasized about confronting the group of porters and guides for their nasty gossiping the night before. I wondered what would have happened if I had run out of my tent in my long johns, the ones that barely covered my butt, and yelled at the lot of them. I wanted to wag my finger, shaming them all for treating me—a paying customer, a person—with such disrespect. "How dare you?" I'd shout, hoping it would shock them into treating me nicely. But I wasn't that brave. Besides, I didn't want to risk giving them more ammunition. Instead, I did what I usually do when it comes to confrontation. I swallowed it, as I swallow everything.

I came back mentally, looked around me, and noticed Stacey and Tracey both looking pale. I asked Tracey how she was doing.

"I'm a little nervous because I feel so queasy. I'm going to try not to focus on it because then I'll feel more sick," she said. "I probably ate something that didn't agree with me."

She didn't want to blame it on the altitude, because that would only get worse as we went higher on the mountain.

Stacey sorted through her backpack: wet wipes, rain gear, snacks, and poles attached to the side of the backpack in case she needed them. I went right to filling up my Camelbak, dropping in iodine tablets and Gatorade mix.

"It's like a dexterity test at this altitude," I said to Stacey as I tried to screw the cap back on. The water pouch wriggled like a fish anytime I tried to secure the top. The Gatorade sloshed out and made my hands sticky. The red liquid ran between my fingers, still grimy from the previous day's hike.

Stacey just gave me a blank stare. I tried to keep her spirits up. Focusing my energy on someone worse off than me made me feel a little better. I didn't want to tell anyone about the previous night's laugh fest. It was already too embarrassing with just me knowing about it.

"I'm trying to keep some electrolytes flowing through my body. I know there are extra calories in there, but we'll be hiking up some high, hard hills for three hours, maybe five," I announced to Stacey, trying to sound a bit like a jock.

I tried to nudge the Camelbak into the slot between the back of the pack and the compartment that housed my notebook, jacket, and sunscreen.

"Shimmy, shimmy," I said, feeling like everyone was watching me, starting to laugh at me. I often looked up and saw people just watching. After the previous evening, I felt like I was entertainment.

I tried to make light of it and hammed it up like the funny fat girl, but it came off like uncomfortable babble. "You know it's funny, yesterday they said I had too many things in my bag, and I realized that I had my journal and my solar charger box and all these extra things. So it's actually a little lighter today."

I had removed those things, kept them in my duffle bag for the porters to carry. I never used any of them. The whole trip, they were just extra weight.

My daypack still weighed about twenty pounds with all the water in it. When we were all finished packing up, we headed up a skinny trail that looped up and around Mawenzi Peak. Getting so close to the jagged rock made me nervous. The steep trail had a long drop below.

A Mawenzi hike is a technical climb, requiring ropes, ice axes, and such. Even if I weighed 120 pounds, I wouldn't be interested in that.

Sally looked up at Kilimanjaro ahead and saw another camp below the peak. "So that's it up there . . . where we are going?"

"Yep. After all we did yesterday, this will be a cakewalk," I said. I didn't believe this because even though this day's hike was shorter, this was steeper. And, it was a higher altitude.

"We have really great scenery on this hike," Sally said. Focusing on the positive was the way she cared for Tracey, who seemed to be dragging a little bit. She looked down queasily at rocks and *Senecio* trees below, which looked like giant matted mops with tufts of green on top. Stacey looked up at the hills as if she was going to hurl. She asked, "So, there are no more peaks once we get up to the top there; we go down to camp, right?"

"No," Kenedy said, pausing, as if wondering if he should have said that. Stacey immediately sank a little. I could see in her slump that she was wondering if she could do this.

"We camp at the base of Mawenzi Peak. I think it's a couple thousand feet up," I said.

"I think it was something like 1,380 feet, at least that's what it said on the paperwork," Sally, who had memorized the itinerary, chimed in.

"How it translates into how we feel today, we'll see," I said.

Stacey looked wistful, hunched over her poles. "I would rather hike feeling queasy than with cramps," she said, looking for the bright side.

I needed to stop the guessing, the calculations in my own mind about the journey ahead. So I said "*Twende*," or "Let's go," in Swahili.

"Just drink plenty of water," Sally said. I got the feeling Sally and I were a tad too perky for Stacey and Tracey.

"This is all we have to do today. Four hours of this. It's easy," I said.

"Finish line in sight," Sally said.

"Yep," I said. We moved forward. Stacey looked like a car with a stalled engine as she tried to get going, to regain her momentum.

I looked up toward the peak and shouted back to Stacey, "I see where we're going and it's a beautiful thing . . . it may not be pretty yet, but it will be beautiful when we get there."

However far I walked, however much I tried to think of other things, the humiliation of last night was there, and it was raw. I was overcompensating by being perky, a cheerleader, even if I would have never made it on a team, let alone be on the top of a pyramid. But being perky and positive was how I usually dealt with everything in public.

I needed to confront Kenedy, but in such a way that he would continue guiding me up the mountain safely. So, when it came time for a water-and-pee break amid an outcropping of rocks, I approached our guide and did what I always do when I'm upset or nervous: I smiled.

I didn't want him to know that his mocking words had made me want to turn back. So there I was swallowing my true feelings, trying to be nice. After all, his job was not an easy one. He was already carrying Tracey's backpack, to help her.

But my cheeks burned. I had always lived with the feeling I couldn't or shouldn't speak up in the face of bullies, or my abuser, or even my father. I was used to swallowing words, like .22 rifle shells. So when it came time to say my words, I nearly choked on the first syllable.

"I want to talk to you about something," I said, interrupting a Swahili conversation he was having with our assistant guide, Michael. "Last night, I heard you. You were talking about me. What were you saying?"

"Sorry?" Kenedy said. I was pretty sure he was pretending he didn't know what I was talking about.

"I heard you last night. I heard you making the noises I make when going up and down the trail. 'Ruh. Ruh. Ruh,'" I said.

"I was talking with some porters who wanted to know, 'Are you sure she's going to make it?' I was answering them. They don't believe you are going to the top," Kenedy said. He looked embarrassed, maybe not because of what he said, but for getting caught.

From his tone the night before, I couldn't help but think that he was one of the people betting against my success. I knew his laughter and believed he laughed at me.

"They don't believe it?" I asked.

"Yeah," Kenedy answered, looking away.

"Did you make any money bets?" I asked. "You should," I said, pausing. "Bet on me. Bet on me."

The words exited my mouth like a bucket of burrs. They stung me on the way out but once they came out, it was a relief, the sweet joy of saying what I felt.

I wasn't going to allow myself to be the joke. I wasn't going to allow anyone to treat me that way. Not anymore. This was it. If I was going to go up the mountain, I needed a guide. I didn't need someone who thought they could hurt me again and again as my abuser did, as my taunters did, as my father did.

But in that moment of confronting Kenedy, I feared deeply that he would leave, run back down the mountain. This vast feeling of emptiness, me on the porch with my father, consumed me. Please don't go. Please don't go. We can't go on without you.

I could see in his face that he was sorry.

"We won't do that again," Michael said.

My body shook a bit as I felt the exchange hanging in the air. But now that it was out there two things needed to happen. I needed to make it up the mountain.

We walked directly toward our new camp for that night. My steps seemed lighter, easier; I felt a power in my movement that I hadn't felt before.

I plunged my poles into the earth and went forward.

I earned a little respect and stood up for myself. There on the rock, I finally talked back instead of eating my feelings. And it was delicious.

As Kenedy and Michael walked ahead, Tracey pulled me aside and scolded me.

"Why did you do that?" Tracey said. She was mad that I confronted the guides when they were already doing so much for us. "Culturally, you do stick out. You call yourself fat. Why was it a problem for someone else to do so?"

I fumed back, "Wouldn't you do that if you were in a restaurant and someone was making fun of you?"

"Did they serve me my meal?"

"Yes. But there they are, humiliating you."

"Then no, I would just eat my meal," she said smugly.

I thought that Tracey was being a total bitch. She seemed to be saying, not only did I deserve to be humiliated, but I asked for it, just by being there on the mountain.

"That's terrible customer service. I wouldn't put up with that, and yes, I would complain," I said, still shaking from the interaction. "That wouldn't bother you? Look, I'm three hundred pounds; people laugh at me all the fucking time. I'm sick of it. I want to prove him wrong. I'm going to prove them wrong."

"I know that you're going to make it to the top, and you know that you're going to make it to the top," Tracey said. "If I were in your shoes, I don't know that I would have confronted him because it wouldn't put me in a better place. It would have made no difference in my ability to make it to the top of that mountain."

"It doesn't make a difference. I just wanted to know if they were saying what I thought they were saying. I just wanted to know," I said, and I didn't want negative talk about me to follow me up the mountain. I had enough of it in my own mind.

What I wanted them to know, most of all, was it hurt.

Maybe Tracey heard the trembling in my voice, because she backed down a bit. "This is just me being an armchair psychologist/drill sergeant," she said, semi-apologetically.

"I made an executive decision to use those Wisps on my teeth. Bad decision," said Stacey, trying to break the tension. She gritted her teeth together and showed how plaque was accumulating along her gums in a big, goofy smile.

Stacey was feeling lousy enough and didn't want to be around negativity from anyone. She just had to get through to the next camp. The conversation ended there but the air between us was still stagnant. Heavy.

Tracey didn't think I did the right thing. I knew that. But for the first time in a very long time I felt like I had.

I made a scene, not by knocking something off a table with my gargantuan hips, but by announcing I wasn't going to put up with that kind of treatment anymore. I said what I needed to say and I was going to be okay.

That moment was for all the people out there who shame others for being fat. I didn't really want to be in this body but I was. There was no need to make it harder for me. Those people expect us to be thinner but then ridicule us when we are working out. You nudge us to have an ice cream sundae, only to give us grief about it later. My words were for them.

Fuck them for trying to make someone bigger feel smaller. They don't know our stories. They don't know that words can eviscerate us despite our thick skin.

I know why it's so hard for people who are my size to be active. You can feel brave and strong, have a date on your calendar to work out, but there is something so vulnerable about putting yourself out there, in sweatpants or spandex, in a world you don't fit in.

Even on this trip, I wavered between believing I was going to make it and feeling destined for failure. The mind can trip itself in an instant, and then all is lost.

Tracey grew increasingly frustrated with me over the course of the day. She walked ahead of me and only talked to Sally. She wished I could believe in myself 100 percent of the time and stop making it so uncomfortable for everyone else.

"Sometimes, if you catch her at just the right moment, you can tell she's still very self-conscious about it," she said to Sally about my weight. She was right. I wanted to walk away from her.

At home, I would have just hung up the phone and called a friend to complain or sent out a passive-aggressive Facebook post. Something like "Some people just don't get it." But here, I was forced to face her. I was forced to face Kenedy. I was forced to face myself.

As the distance between us grew larger, I thought maybe I should have backed down. Maybe I should have let things lie and apologize to both Tracey and Kenedy. But if I didn't say anything, it just would have festered, creating an even bigger distance between us. I wanted to talk with Stacey, but she could only muster the energy to walk.

I found myself searching for a Clif Bar, something to tamp down the sting of the confrontation. But I came up empty and I didn't want to heave off my backpack just to nosh.

My heart beat faster. My chest tightened. My mind raced.

"Alright guys, *twende*," Michael said, trying to break the chill that had descended between us and get us hiking back to full speed, which was more like a two out of ten on a treadmill.

I immediately leapt into cheerleader mode.

"Okay, guys, do you have it in you for one more incline today?" I turned to Michael. "You can do it. How do you say, 'You can do it' in Swahili?"

"*Unaweza*," he repeated back to me and pointed to the path ahead.

"*Unaweza*," I said back and he nodded.

Unaweza became my mantra, cycling through my head up hills, down hills, and around the bends. I said it to myself, trying to drown out the swishing of my pants' thighs rubbing together.

I took my poles in one hand to put my other hand on a rock, gingerly thudding down on the ground below me. As much as the mantra helped me, I couldn't escape the fact that we were trudging along at 12,000 feet where I found less and less oxygen to breath.

My head started to tingle. Then pain bore into my skull.

But with each step, the scope of my headache widened. I could see Mawenzi Tarn Camp, an oasis of tents surrounding a mountain lake in the distance. We had been walking six hours to get there and it was just over a stream and a small hill in the landscape. But I wasn't sure I could make it.

At first, I tried to push the headache away. I feel fine, I told myself. I'll be alright. But words weren't enough. I saw the camp ahead and tried to take longer steps, to get there faster. But by exerting myself, I just made the pain in my head worse.

Then, as I stepped down from a rock, I felt dizzy. I was losing my grip.

I had some pain reliever in my pocket, and it was time to take it. Maybe that would solve the problem. But I knew that at this height, I was no longer in control of my body. I tore open the packet, then immediately dropped it, watching as it fluttered down in the air like a butterfly.

I moaned as I leaned down to grab it, stretching my hamstrings in a way that felt unexpectedly amazing. Then, in an instant, all the blood rushed down to my head so suddenly that I nearly toppled over, and the dizziness continued as I straightened up. The sand-colored rocks spun around me. I had to put my hand on the rock wall to stop the motion. Steadying myself, I popped the pill and swallowed it down with a Gatorade-iodine cocktail.

We passed a rock cairn, the kind where people stack rocks on top of each other, and it kind of looked like me—big on the bottom and skinny on top. It was a statue of sorts, or maybe an homage to my shape, as if I belonged there.

I thought of that as I made my way along the winding trail, bordered by yellow wildflowers sprouting amid the moss, the first flora I'd seen in several hours. I wobbled uneasily on the increasingly difficult trail. The wind started to pick up, and we were within its current, ebbing and flowing. To our left, we could see patches of Kenya below.

"Isn't that so cool, the clouds being right there? You can only see that in an airplane," I said.

My brain felt squeezed as if my skull was in a vice. Fortunately, my pain meds were kicking in, so I was able to put on a good face when I arrived at camp even though I was the last one. I didn't want anyone to know how much my head hurt. "This is easy-peasy. Camp three and I still have a smile on my face," I announced, hoping a porter, one who wasn't part of my conversation with Kenedy, would hear me. But there were none around. Really, I was talking to myself.

Didn't they see me on the mountain, trying hard? Couldn't they appreciate how difficult this was for me? Instead of mocking me, couldn't they appreciate the effort it took for me to just be there?

"I'm just going to rest for a little bit," I said, heading to my tent. I climbed in, closed the zipper, and started to cry.

My head, which had felt better for a while, started to hurt again. My self-esteem felt torn. My façade was breaking.

I just wanted to be home and comfortable.

I lifted my hands over my face. Every little crevice on every finger was covered in dirt, as if my hands were a map. The tips of my fingernails were black, like a reverse French manicure. I pulled my nail file out of my bag and tried to clean my hands, but it only seemed to push the dirt in deeper.

I'm disgusting, I thought, as one of the porters dropped a pail of water outside my tent for washing up. I fumbled through my duffle bag to find a washcloth and dunked it into the lukewarm water, which felt good and refreshing. It made me feel better for the moment.

I pulled the washcloth across my forehead, making a clean streak amidst dirt. Each swath of the washcloth made a new streak. When I dunked the washcloth back in, the water immediately turned brown.

I continued the same routine with my arms, adding in peppermint backpacker's soap, which had been with me all three trips. I tried to get clean but only seemed to add the same dirt back onto myself. I rolled up my pant legs, only to find my calves and inner pant legs covered in dirt. I looked like the chimney sweep scene in Mary Poppins and smelled like a giant muddy mint. I took off my sock and saw there was a definitive line marking the difference between my clean foot and dirty leg.

As I flexed my foot to clean the sole, I saw a defined calf muscle.

"Boom," I thought to myself. It was no six-pack but I was getting stronger, even if no one else could tell.

I needed to bet on me, too.

CHAPTER 24

Self-Medicating

DAY 3: AFTERNOON,
MAWENZI TARN CAMP, 14,206 FEET

INSTEAD OF MEETING AT THE dining tent for a snack, we went in shifts. I was glad to have the solitude, to be alone with my tea and popcorn.

We had a few moments of downtime before a short acclimatization hike up the trail, to help us get used to being above 15,000 feet—because four hours of hiking just wasn't enough. Just the thought of it made my head pound.

As I slurped my tea and crunched my popcorn, the sounds echoed in my head like a giant's steps through this beautiful open setting, as if the camp were about to be taken over and destroyed.

I clutched my head quietly, hoping no one would notice, rubbing my temples. Pushing firmly in and rotating, I tried to distract myself from the dark creeping in.

I found my yellow tent and flopped down inside. This wasn't a pop-a-Tylenol-and-be-done-with-it headache. It was one that bore deep into my skull and radiated through my body.

We had time in our little tents to soak in what was bothering us. Sally hated being covered in dirt. It was everywhere: her hair, her clothing, her backpack. Still, she tried to make a Buff headscarf fashionable. When she smiled, the dirt highlighted every little crinkle in her face, from the crow's-feet that accentuated her eyes to her dimpled cheeks.

Tracey hated feeling unsure about whether or not she was going to have trouble breathing.

Stacey hated feeling ill and excused herself from the acclimatization hike to rest. She tried to clean up at camp using her dry shampoo but it only made her hair clumpy and feel dirtier.

I was left alone with a headache that would not go away. I wanted to will myself to forget it. But it was there, the pounding getting stronger every minute.

"I feel fine," I whispered to myself over and over.

When Michael came to my tent to say it was time for the acclimatization hike, I figured I'd walk it off. But as we started up over the jagged teeth of Mawenzi, my head throbbed on, feeling as heavy as if someone had hung an anvil around my neck.

About 800 feet into this 1,200-foot jaunt, I couldn't take another step. Sally and Tracey were in front of me, and I quietly told Michael that I needed to go back to my tent. The camp below looked like a play set.

He could see by my glazed eyes that I was not well. He told one of the porters to go along with me.

A severe headache could be a sign of cerebral edema. If that was the case, my choice to go down would be pretty clear. Still, as I saw the others making their way up to a vista, away from me, I was jealous and embarrassed that I wasn't with them. I was retreating when there was work to be done. But I had to rest. I had to listen to my body.

The sun beat down on my tent, shining through my eyelids. I covered my face with my arm, not at all sure how I was going to get up in the morning and do this for another day.

I inhaled deeply, then reached for my altitude medication, dexamethasone—a small dose of steroid meant to reduce inflammation.

I typically wasn't much into pharmaceuticals, although I did seem to get plenty of food fixes at CVS and drugstores. Call it self-medicating.

I found myself in the candy aisles between maple nut goodies and cara-mel chews every time I was there to pick up something else, whether it was diapers or laundry detergent. Make a good decision today, I'd think. Even if I put something back, I often picked up something new—a Twix bar or a box of cookies—in the checkout aisle.

I wondered if people in the security viewing area could see me. I wondered if they laughed at me and my obsessive traipsing back and forth from aisle to aisle.

Once, a doctor in Vermont put me on Prozac to help me lose weight. Another time, at my request, another doctor put me on Meridia for the same reason. Neither really worked, or I should say, I never really worked to make it a success. The pills may have curbed my physical appetite but I still ate crap, even if I wasn't hungry, even if I felt a little happier.

Happiness wasn't my problem. Sadness was. It was locked down deep below all my layers. I had turned my body into a catacomb contain-ing bad memories.

I wished there was a castor oil–like drug that would help me purge the memories and be done with them, once and for all. I wanted a Mr. Creosote moment from Monty Python's *The Meaning of Life*, retching all my bad memories up in buckets and buckets until they were gone. If only it were that easy.

For me, chocolate worked better than antidepressants to rebalance my serotonin, or so I told myself.

But I had a habit of overloading my circuits. After that first bite, that first peak, I wanted to keep going, to float there, forever. But it doesn't work that way. After the first few surges, it all comes to a crashing halt, down to the floor with the empty bag, the crumpled foil wrappers.

I WAS THE LAST IN our group to start the altitude medication. Sally, Sta-cey, and Tracey had been on it since we'd arrived at the first camp. The Diamox made their fingers feel tingly. It also made them pee every few hours, since the drug's job is to flush the system.

Diamox is a sulfa-based drug, and since I'm allergic to it, I had to go for the alternative, dexamethasone. But because it's a steroid, you have to use it sparingly, to wait until you can't stand the symptoms anymore, or else the drug itself can make you crazy, hyper, a complete madwoman.

After I caved and gave myself a dose, I'd need to repeat it every six hours until the summit.

I was also taking the herb gingko biloba, known in climbing circles as a natural way to acclimatize. I'd been popping the clear capsules for two weeks. It was supposed to be a natural blood thinner, helping to prevent the danger of embolism. I had read that giving up caffeine could help make acclimatization easier. So in the weeks before the trek, I slowly weaned myself off coffee.

Giving up caffeine was okay, because while some people use coffee as a calorie-free appetite suppressant, for me it often ended up being a means to a different end. Instead of drinking it black, or with skim milk, I'd order up caramel swirl-this or mocha-frappé-that.

Whipped-cream Frappuccinos left a film inside my mouth that was both satisfying and scary. Sometimes, I would imagine the stuff lining my arteries. That didn't stop me from ordering another. Leave it to me to turn what could be a zero-calorie beverage into four hundred liquid calories.

The biggest trouble with coffee was that it makes me feel anxious and sets off a roller coaster of uneasy emotions that inevitably lifts me out of my chair to find something—anything (a graham cracker, a banana)—to anchor me. Then comes the sugar crash. I'd feel tired, so I'd reach for another cup of coffee. Then I'd repeat the cycle (between trips to the bathroom).

I hoped this tiny little dexamethasone tablet would get me through, give me just enough of an edge so I could make it to the top and back down, victorious. I closed my eyes and waited.

CHAPTER 25

Fresh Start

DAY 4: SUNRISE, MAWENZI TARN CAMP, 14,206 FEET

When I opened my eyes the next day, I immediately knew. My head was better. The day before, my eyes watered from the pain. The dried tears had soaked up the dirt that was crusted in my eyelashes. I took a slow breath of relief. I'd made it through the night. I could continue on. I would be okay, for today anyway.

I knew it was morning by the glow in my tent and the sounds of the porters and guides setting up for the day. The clinking of pots and mumbling of Swahili had become my cue to wake up. I didn't want to waste my cell phone battery since my solar charger was kaput, so I decided to gauge what time it was by stepping outside my tent.

It was a gorgeous day. Brilliant blue sky framed the tawny brown mountains that waved like an ocean around us. This was the peace I had been waiting for. This was the beauty I needed to see and feel within me.

When I stood up, my powder-gray hiking pants sagged around my waist. Back home, they had clung to my hips with no fabric to spare. Now, I had to hold them up with a bootlace. After all, I didn't want to moon anyone on summit night.

Tying the lace in a knot, I smiled a cocky little smile at myself. It felt good to be losing inches. To be carving fat off my body and letting go of pounds and grief I was holding on to.

Still, I didn't want to be too confident. We had three more days of full-tilt hiking to reach the top, and then get down safely.

I put on my wool hat and long-sleeved shirt and joined the group for breakfast.

Our water bottles were lined up next to the dining tent, ready for us. In the previous days, the porters were able to gather our water from fresh sources. Here, at the third camp, they could only pull it from a stagnant high-altitude pond.

I had been over to that mossy, green water source the previous day. I tried not to think about what it looked and smelled like as I dropped iodine and Gatorade into my bottle, making a swirling mud smoothie. The porters would have to carry enough water from this source to Kibo Hut, where we would launch our summit attempt. We needed it to survive. Except none of us wanted anything to do with the swill.

After the previous day, I felt compelled to clear the air, to focus on the day ahead, and to get us through. We all had our own agenda. Mine was to finish on top—mentally and physically. Stacey's to honor her parents. Sally and Tracey's to train for the IMAZ.

I walked over to the breakfast table to find them all slumped over steaming bowls of gruel and fruit. If there was ever a time for a pep talk, this was it.

I sat down for a moment, but then sprang off my bucket, which returned to its proper form, and stood at the head of the table as if I were making a toast at some formal dinner party.

"Imagine, less than twenty-four hours from now, we'll all be on top of the mountain. It will be hard, but it's just a day," I said. "It's such a gorgeous day. We've had terrific weather the whole way through. You have no idea how great that is. My water bottle didn't freeze so that means it's not too cold." I was rambling now.

They looked up, squinting as the sun rose higher in the sky.

"You have all been such an inspiration to me. Sally, you have been so positive. Tracey, you didn't feel great, but you pushed on. Stacey, oh my God, you lost it and came back again. Right now it's about 8:00 AM. In twenty-four hours you will be standing on the summit of Kilimanjaro. So, it may be the most difficult day of your entire life. It might be the most grueling, the most painful, and the dirtiest, but it's just one day. Just remember that to get through it."

I nodded to Sally. "You've been dreaming about this for ten years, and the moment is here," I said.

I addressed Sally and Tracey, "And I know you've been working toward this for years. Every day you made yourself go to the gym or made a good decision that pays off here. This is what you've worked for and I am so proud of you all. You have no idea how well you are doing.

"If we can just give it everything, we're going to get there. I promise. Just pole, pole—slowly, slowly, and we'll get there. So, yay. Go team Kili!"

I looked down at the table and saw everyone crying.

"I'm sorry. I didn't mean to get you all weepy," I said, sitting back down.

"I can't believe in twenty-four hours . . . " Sally said. For a decade she had hoped to have the time, money, and opportunity to be on this mountain, and here she was.

Tracey turned to her. "You're making me cry. Ten years you've been waiting for this, and I am so happy to be here with you."

They grabbed each other's hands. "And I'm going to make it," Sally said.

"You are," Tracey said.

There was still a desire to look and feel good on the mountain in the darkest of moments. We wanted to make sure our shirts were tucked in, our hair was pulled back, and our backpacks had our sunscreen and water for the day. Those were the little things we could hold on to, to make us feel good, to make us feel ready for the last big push to summit camp. We were a little more bundled up than yesterday, as the temperature hovered at about thirty-five degrees. Our water bottles didn't freeze but it felt cold enough for us to freeze. I ducked back in my tent for my hat and gloves.

Tracey fixed Sally's headband, an orange swath of cloth that also worked as a mask to keep the dust out of her mouth. "You look very '50s mod."

Sally turned toward Stacey and me. "Do I?"

"Very cute," Stacey said, smiling a little. She was still being quiet, but looking better than she had the past few days. She had color in her cheeks again. "And I'm getting my appetite back," Stacey said. "I never thought I'd hear myself say I lost my appetite."

"High altitude is a funny thing," I said, laughing and handing Stacey her Camelbak. I hoped pumping her up mentally would help her physically.

"I'm just nervous that I'm not going to make it," she said. She had been constantly calculating travel and rest times in her head. She needed to set aside eight hours to rest with Ambien. So on each day, we had to get to the next camp with plenty of time to spare, we needed to trek faster in the higher altitude. Otherwise, she worried she would get almost no sleep and be physically wiped out for the rest of the trek. She had a lingering headache and continued trouble eating; also she tended to ramble.

"I'll get through today and if I feel better I'll attempt the summit no matter what," Stacey said. "I want to do it, but I don't want to feel like shit and do it. I guess it just comes with not feeling good. And I haven't been eating . . . a couple of bites here and there, but I know I'm going to need the energy to get up there. I don't know if I'm going to be able to have the energy to get there.

"Physically, I could do it. If I could get eight hours of sleep," Stacey continued. The only thing that was holding her back was her appetite. The only thing she could stomach was Clif Bars. "I'd rather be at the top, ready to come down. I'm not going to let a headache stop me. If I have to eat twenty Clif Bars instead of the food that they serve, that's what I'll do."

For her, this trip wasn't just a hike; it was becoming a nightmare. It had become a punishing journey that ripped out her insides and told her to keep marching regardless.

"Today's going to be flat, right?" Stacey asked.

"All we have to do is clear that bend over there and go straight across the Saddle," I said, pointing to a vista that looked no bigger than a hill in my hometown of Summit. It looked like an incline I'd need to walk a bike up, but I could get up it. But I warned her that just because a section looked flat did not mean that it would be easy.

The Saddle part of the trek, especially, was a mind game. Once you cleared a few inclines, it looked like a straightforward walk to the camp, but we were about to enter desert terrain, a barren stretch that would make our current mountain camp seem like an oasis.

No matter how far you hike over this terrain, the summit peak doesn't seem to get any closer. It's flat and you're hiking at an altitude higher than most of the Rocky Mountains. But we had put ourselves on the mountain for a reason. It wasn't just for charity. We could have just asked folks to contribute without hiking the mountain. Climbing the mountain was for us. As the summit loomed, there seemed to be increased pressure to get it right, to accomplish our missions.

We got up from the table and went to collect our stuff; we could tell the porters were anxious to get going. Once they arrived at the next camp, most of them would be off for a day. They would meet up with dozens of other porters from other trekking companies, seeing old friends and comparing notes. I kind of dreaded that, knowing I would likely be a topic of conversation.

The day's hike would start straight uphill, ascending like a roller coaster—up, up, and up—so we could go down the other side and across the Saddle, straight on to our summit attempt.

I steadied myself by reaching out my gloved hand and placing it on a rock, constantly balancing between hiking poles and the nearly ver- tical ground. Even Sally was having trouble walking. Every few steps exhausted her. None of us could do as well as the porters, who were facing the incline with grace and speed.

Instead, each step was tentative, to be sure the next wouldn't end in a broken ankle.

As we reached the top of the ridge, the view stopped us in our tracks. Suddenly, it was just us and the mountaintop.

The previous day it had dodged in and out of view. Now, here it was in all its splendor. This was, indeed, the final approach.

CHAPTER 26

Crumbling

DAY 4: MAWENZI TARN CAMP, 14,330 FEET

"One hand here. One foot there. One foot here," I said, carefully making it down the rocks. One rock wobbled and fell below me. I watched it go, imagining all three hundred pounds of me tumbling down the ridge on the way to the Saddle. "This time I might actually break the rocks." The rocks felt fragile, unstable, and so did I.

"You got it," Stacey said, also looking down to steady herself.

"Once we get past these rocks, we'll be okay," I said.

On the way to Mawenzi Tarn Camp, the rocky trek had started to feel less like a hike and more like a forced march, not least because we were doing it at 14,000 feet. Plus, three hundred pounds is three hundred pounds, even if you're holding hiking sticks or sporting sturdy boots. On the mountain, I carry it all with me. Every ounce.

"I feel we're on the longest walk of our lives," Stacey said.

All I could manage was "Yeah."

Our steps made a distinct noise. Scratch, plunk. Scratch, plunk. Scratch, plunk. The scenery didn't matter anymore. All that consumed us was the sound of our steps. We looked only at the ground, at our own feet. Welcome to Kilimanjaro's Saddle, a plateau connecting Mawenzi and Kilimanjaro.

Scratch, plunk. Scratch, plunk. Scratch, plunk.

It rained very little during our weeklong trek, which was great for keeping us dry. But it also meant the mountain was dry, and with each step we kicked up the earth. For protection from the dust, we pulled our bandanas over our faces. I could tell by Stacey's eyes, which squinted behind her sunglasses, that she needed another break. I reminded her, "The slower you hike, the better."

But at this point, I felt like she was going to punch me. She was sick of my pep talks.

Sally and Tracey were racers; they perpetually moved forward, even when Stacey and I stopped to rest. Our one group became two, leaving Stacey and me with each other.

Stacey and I were family. We were both fat. This gave her the right and privilege to hate me (temporarily). Even if she was a hundred pounds lighter than I, we had the same beast of burden. Stacey and I made excuses for each other. We were the ones feeling our extra weight in our knees, in our backs, absorbing the gawking, which in itself was a big load to bear.

But it helped to bear it together. It was great to have someone who got it. We were both hungry for something. We were hungry for love, past or present. We both ate to fill an emptiness—for me, the void my father left; for her, the untimely loss of her parents.

Like old guys gathered in a bar, we would be the two ordering the super-sweet Frappuccinos, or stopping for happy hour hors d'oeuvres together, bonding with food.

Unfortunately, with Stacey bent over with stomach cramps from the altitude and not getting any better, I had to go slow to accommodate her. I have to admit, at my size and with the blisters burning through my heel and right big toe, it felt better to go slow.

I just knew we were in the same boat. I had inspired her to do this and now here she was, doing it. I couldn't step out of that limelight. Everything I did mattered. I felt responsible for her.

"I thought this was supposed to be the plateau. I thought that was the last hill," she said.

I leaned on my poles, trying to ignore her. I didn't want to look tired so I pretended to stretch to catch a break. The questions reminded me of my daughter's constant road trip chimes of "Are we there yet?"

We eventually caught up to Sally and Tracey, who seemed to be enjoying a rest, leaning on their hiking poles.

Stacey turned to Kenedy for an answer: "Is this the last steep part?"

He just nodded, although we both weren't sure if it was really true.

"I'm going to hold you to that," Stacey said.

"She might beat you up if it isn't," Sally joked.

Stacey and I borrowed the language of my spinning instructor.

Slow. Steady. Strong. With each step we tried to overcome our internal dialogue telling us the trail was never going to end.

"Are these switchbacks like the ones on the summit climb?" Stacey asked, looking up to see a maze of them up ahead.

"Sort of," I answered. I didn't want to tell her that she had scree, a surface that slides underfoot, to look forward to. If this was hard, that was going to be ten times harder.

We arrived at the top of the ridge and cheered, which seems silly in hindsight when the real challenge would be traversing 800 more feet of mountain in front of us. Still, it was a victory that needed to be honored.

"I'M ACTUALLY HUNGRY. I COULD eat a Clif Bar," Stacey said.

"Do it, do it," I cheered.

"I have like fifteen if you need extra," she said. "I thought I would be eating like three a day."

"I knew you would rally. You've been through so much already," I said, passing yellow flowers billowing in the breeze. It was a bit of a surprise to find them so high up where rock and cloud were all I could see.

"I didn't come all this way to crap out . . . literally," she said.

We both roared with laughter. It had been days since I'd seen Stacey smile.

CHAPTER 27

Wreckage

DAY 4: THE SADDLE, 15,000 FEET—NOONISH

THE SADDLE BETWEEN MAWENZI AND Kilimanjaro's peak was like a lonely dusty road in the Old West. There were rocks the size of bowling balls strewn randomly on either side of the path. Every now and then a cloud whispered by, hiding the peak or the path ahead. It enveloped us, then left.

The alpine desert was bare, empty, and ugly. Nothing but sand in every direction—apart from the life and flora at the bottom of the mountain and the glory of the mountaintop. However, in order to succeed, we had to go through it.

We were exposed in every way. Every now and then there was a gust of wind but nothing to hold on to except for a few scattered boulders. The sun beat on us as if we were ants under a magnifying glass since we were 15,000 feet closer to it than at home. SPF 100 didn't feel like enough.

We had been marching on the seemingly never-ending stretch for six hours. In the distance, we saw what looked like a downed airplane.

We walked toward it, painfully, slowly, until we could clearly see bits of it scattered over the mountain. Michael told us that a couple paid a pilot to get a closer glimpse of Kilimanjaro. They all perished. In the years since the crash had happened, no one had carried the twisted metal remains off the mountainside. There it stayed as a monument to what happened.

The wreckage seemed like a bad omen. As a journalist, I was used to focusing on the worst that could happen.

My first day working at the *Ventura County Star* in California, a man led police on a high-speed car chase into Simi Valley, to an intersection where an eighty-year-old man was waiting patiently at the stoplight in his convertible. The old man was the type who ate oranges every day, and took care of his wife who had a heart condition. He loved his four daughters. And in an instant, the high-speed runaway struck his vehicle from behind, sending it skyward. It landed upside down. The old man was killed.

I had to tell his story. The night after I wrote it, I went to Trader Joe's, then went home and stuffed myself sick before falling asleep on my air mattress in a rented room. All I could see was the upside-down car surrounded with police tape.

Over the years, I became good at telling other people's tragic stories with compassion and care. In fact, I was often the go-to person on staff when it came to confronting the human side of tragedy.

"Tell me about your son," I'd say. "Tomorrow there will be a story about his death, and I want to focus on his life."

I really felt that way. It meant sitting through funerals and wakes for people I'd never met. I reported on dozens of central New Jersey September 11 victims; a woman raped by assailants who bashed her skull in with a cinderblock; children killed by their mother, who blamed it on a cocktail of Prozac, wine, and her cheating husband; and a cheerleader who dropped in the middle of practice and later died because of a glitch in her heart.

I told all these stories with detail and a sense of duty and rarely cried. After all, that wouldn't be professional. I spent a decade as a journalist, but after I was laid off, I decided it was the perfect opportunity to step away from it. I didn't need to immerse myself in sadness and tragedy. My profession, moving forward, was to stay healthy.

As I looked at the wreckage, I thought about the people trying to get a quick glimpse of something that normally takes days to see. Maybe they couldn't hike the mountain themselves and this was their only way up? It was supposed to be the easy route, but it was over before they could go home.

Life in itself is dangerous. You could be killed coming home from work. You could make the wrong move and find yourself under a falling object. You could be out shopping and get carjacked.

If there was anything that my journalism career taught me, it was how to live. Nevertheless, it was easier for me to live by dulling my pain with food.

I was usually twisted up with anxiety, my brain churning through nightmare scenario after nightmare scenario. If I heard sirens down the street, I worried that my daughter had been hurt at daycare. If I glimpsed a giant tree limb, I couldn't help thinking it might fall on me.

Sally had been a journalist for decades, beginning in her twenties. She was a traffic reporter known as "Sally in the Sky." It inspired her to learn to fly planes, just like the one smashed to bits on the mountain. Over the years she became more grounded and found her passion as a national television reporter.

"Yeah, after so many murders, carjackings, and children going missing or getting killed—and plane crashes like this—it does take a toll," Sally said.

My past as a journalist translated into me being an über-cautious mother. If there was a pool nearby, I held my child tightly at all times because of all the drownings I'd covered.

And if I should ever have any inclination that there might be a gun in a house, my kid won't be allowed there. These fears were based on things that happened to a small percentage of people, but they were very real to me. I knew you could get killed chopping down a tree in your backyard. I knew you could get killed walking across the street.

"Or driving to work," Sally said.

"Driving to work," I echoed. "Every day you are faced with risks and challenges and you never know when it's your time. I know I'm well trained for this journey. I wouldn't put myself up here if I wasn't, because the second time I didn't make it and I felt very afraid for my life. But this time I feel ready." I really did feel safe.

"Life can get you any day . . . and it got these people on that day. They probably thought they were just on vacation and were going to take some beautiful photos and be back on their way," I said.

"It's true," Sally said. "But there is danger involved in what we're doing. There is risk."

"On that note, I'll be taking my dexamethasone," I said.

"Yeah," Sally said.

We passed the pieces of fuselage and shards of twisted metal, trying to put it behind us. We would soon arrive at our camp at Kibo Hut. After an early dinner and a short rest, we would be on our way to the summit. None of us knew whether Stacey would be joining us. Each one of her steps was dragging as if she couldn't take another. I thought she had recovered but she was fighting illness again. Sally and Tracey pushed through, as if they were pushing through mile eleven of a half marathon.

CHAPTER 28

Burning Nipples

DAY 4: THE SADDLE, 15,000 FEET

"Drink. Drink the whole thing," I commanded Stacey.

We'd been hiking for seven hours, and Stacey hadn't had more than a half liter of water. She looked at the bottle I held out as if it were battery acid. She was typically strong and stoic despite her ailments. She now looked limp, defeated.

"No," Tracey said. "She'll get sick if she guzzles the whole thing. Little sips, Stacey."

"Chug it. You need that water now," I said, thrusting it at her. I was mad. Mad and tired. Quite honestly, I was pissed that she wasn't taking care of herself. Here we were, in the middle of the Saddle, an alpine desert that looked like something out of *Mad Max Beyond Thunderdome*. Unfortunately, the only vehicle to transport us here was our own, increasingly blistered feet.

"Take five sips," I relented.

She pushed the bottle back down. "I'm not your three-year-old," she said, rolling her eyes.

After four days of being the group cheerleader, I was turning into a bit of a dictator. I needed my hiking mates to start caring for themselves, mostly because I wasn't sure if I could take care of myself, let alone them.

When Stacey mentioned my daughter, I teared up. I missed Anna terribly. The past days of endless stepping, thinking of myself and my family, I'd come to face the rising feeling that over the years, especially in the beginning, I hadn't been fully present with Anna. Was I on the mountain to run away? Was I just as bad as my father, absent even though I was physically there, using food to block really feeling and seeing what she was doing each day?

BEING A NEW MOTHER MADE me understand why good people do bad things to babies, especially at 4:00 AM. I would rock my infant daughter with my bare, crusty feet on the frigid wood floor of our condo, trying to get her to sleep—for the fifth time that night. Life with a colicky four-month-old was hell.

I had worn the same breast milk–stained shirt for days. I hadn't slept a full night—or even a three-hour stretch—in four months. My daughter wailed like a car alarm every time I tried to put her down. So I spent my days with a Boppy nursing pillow around my waist just letting her feed. I felt trapped in the house, my nipples burning.

It wasn't like I was going to hurt my daughter. If it had ever come to that point, I think I would have known to hand her over to someone who could help. I just understood why people would be driven to do such a thing.

I wondered if my overeating while she was in utero made her ravenous, even though she came out a perfect seven pounds ten ounces. One morning, after checking her diaper, rocking her for hours, and still hearing her cries, I was sure I had ruined her before she was even old enough to lift a spoon to her mouth.

I felt it was my fault she was fussy, so I would have to suffer through it alone. I mean, she wouldn't be crying like this as a high school senior, would she?

Would she?!

In the meantime, my sleep-deprived mind couldn't find a solution to her crying. I was on maternity leave, collecting 60 percent of my puny newspaper reporter's salary, and had no money to hire help. Being Anna's mother was my job. And it was the hardest job I'd ever had. Anna got us kicked out of Baby and Me Yoga class because she just would not stop crying, no matter how many times I bounced on the exercise ball with her.

"This used to work with my daughter," the instructor said, perplexed by Anna's roaring.

I'd done prenatal yoga in this studio every Saturday morning during my pregnancy; it was one of the only things that made me feel good during that uncomfortable time. I loved the studio's heated floors that warmed my feet and the way hormones poured through my body as I went through the poses, making me more flexible. In my wide-angle bend, I could reach past the floor almost a foot behind me. Each class would end with a Sanskrit blessing for the babies in our bellies, "*Ohm ma pari man. Oooh maa-ha pari man. Ohm ma-pari man,*" and a gathering with ginger tea and Morning Glory muffins.

The reality of doing baby yoga with an actual infant was more like a nightmare. After taking thirty minutes to bundle up Anna and our things in the car, I spent the time in class trying to ignore dirty looks from the other mothers. Finally, the instructor dismissed us: "Perhaps you can come back and try another time."

So I bundled Anna up again and headed back out into the cold. She fell asleep as soon as she was in her car seat. That's when I started bawling, with my forehead on the steering wheel. I felt rejected. I never went back. I let my six weeks of prepaid classes, $100 of my only expendable income that month, expire.

Instead, I tried to take walks in the neighborhood, hoping to soothe my daughter to sleep. As I wheeled her past neighbors in their fancy yoga pants that clung to their tight asses, they'd say, "That's a hunger cry."

"I just fed her," I'd say. What I was thinking was, Fuck you.

In those rare moments when someone peeked into the carriage and Anna was sleeping, she'd inevitably say, "Aw, this is the Golden Age."

That's when I really wanted to punch someone in the face.

The baby books said a newborn should only nurse every two hours. In those first few months, it felt as if there were only two hours a day when my daughter wasn't at my breast. After being in my belly for nine months, she didn't want to let go. Chris—who seemed to have an inhuman ability to sleep through Anna's wailing—came into the nursery one morning, which was once my office, and asked, "How did she sleep last night?"

I craved my husband's sympathy. I wished I could ask him for comfort. Instead, I raged.

"Sleep?! There was no sleep!" Then I added snidely, "For me, anyway."

Instead of talking to my sweet husband in a normal tone of voice, all I could do was vent and nag. He turned up the heat and came back into the room, still in his T-shirt and boxer shorts. "Want me to change her diaper?"

"Nah, I got it," I said tersely, since Anna was already on the changing table. I flipped open the box of wipes with an exhausted sigh, loud enough for him to hear. Without a word, he left the room to take a shower.

The sound of the shower pissed me off. I wondered if I would get a chance to take one that day. That week. I wondered if our upstairs neighbors would call Child Protective Services if I left Anna wailing in her crib for a few minutes while I stepped outside to breathe.

I walked around the house, bouncing Anna on my hip. If I kept moving, she might stay quiet long enough for Chris to read the newspaper. I wished I could read the newspaper, but every time I sat down to nurse, I seemed to forget it across the room, and I didn't want to risk disturbing the baby. Instead, I watched television.

After my husband left for work, I'd look with scorn at the cereal box he'd leave out on the counter.

Does he think I have nothing to do all day but pick up after him, too? Doesn't he know I work the night shift? What the fuck have I gotten myself into with this baby thing?

My only social outlet was a weekly nursing group, where both the babies and the mothers cried over breast milk. The lactation consultants were often stern with me, reminding me that if I were to dare supplement with formula, I'd lose my own milk supply. "Oh, and by the way," they'd say, "breast milk prevents obesity in your baby's life."

I couldn't bear the thought of my child struggling with obesity. On the other hand, my mother had nursed me for a full year, and I was fat. My husband's mom used formula from the time he was a few weeks old and he was a normal size. Go figure.

I'd return home, balancing my wailing baby in one arm, and using the other hand to open the cereal box flaps and plunge my hand inside. Crunch, crunch, crunch.

It was the only sound I could hear over Anna's screams.

Crunch, crunch, crunch.

I scooped my hand back in to continue this bliss, the sweet and textured grains soothing my soul.

Crunch, crunch, crunch, crunch.

Anna continued to wail for my breast. She couldn't get enough. Crunch. Crunch.

I couldn't either.

CHAPTER 29

Cloud Camp

DAY 4: KIBO HUT CAMP, 15,580 FEET—AFTERNOON

WHILE MOST OF THE TRAIL had been a long, arduous, but generally gentle slope, the rest of Kilimanjaro stood before us like a wall. We were so close that we could no longer see the summit. Everything from the next camp was straight up—the trails zigzagging to help us bear the steep incline. The final steps into camp were the same slog, but all we could focus on was the behemoth before us.

Stacey and I brought up the rear, as usual, while Sally and Tracey went ahead with Kenedy.

I watched as they walked up a hill leading to what looked like an out-of-place summer camp, especially because it had started to snow. Little, light flecks fell from the clouds around our shoulders.

Porters in red and black checked flannel jackets came to get us. This time, they insisted on taking our backpacks. I gladly handed mine over. I wondered if I would have to carry Stacey the rest of the way or hand her off to someone to take her down the mountain.

I was feeling a little lightheaded from the lack of oxygen, and needed someone else to step in to care for Stacey. I didn't feel capable anymore. I needed to care for myself. After consuming about a liter of water, Stacey insisted she was fine to make it to camp. Michael walked a step behind her in case she toppled over. I planted my hiking poles firmly in the ground to make sure I wouldn't do the same.

Our feet scuffed on the ground, but instead of dust, the terrain was more frozen, granular. It felt like one of the first days of winter— cold but not to the point where you would find yourself shivering. A few flakes of snow landed on my fleece jacket and the rocks that jutted around our orange, yellow, and red tents. I wondered what else the sky had in store for us.

I could see the oxygen tank waiting at our campsite. It had been carried up the other side of the mountain by another climbing group that opted for a steeper, shorter way to the top. Knowing it was there felt good, especially because we hadn't needed it the first four days.

Without the backpack, the final steps of the seemingly never-ending hike to Kibo Hut Camp felt effortless.

Other hikers were coming up from the Marangu Route on the eastern side of the mountain. The trails merged for the final ascent. After our days on the remote Rongai Route, the company of other hikers was jarring, even if it amounted to a total of fifteen tents crowded around the last flat stretch of land before a straight uphill incline. I was starting to feel tired and anxious. My insecurities crept back up.

Our camp was one of the first off the trail, so it was easy to duck right into the dining tent, where dinner was set with everything ready, including my bucket. Stacey didn't bother with the dinner tent, heading right into her own tent.

Sally, Tracey, and I took our places around the table, all of us staring blankly, exhausted, none of us knowing what the night would bring. I looked at Stacey's empty place and wondered if it was a sign that she was already gone from this journey—that she was out.

"Think it will keep snowing?" we asked Kenedy and Michael.

"Can't say," Kenedy said.

It was hard enough to lift my legs with no impediments. I hadn't planned on trudging through a foot of snow on an almost vertical slope.

For days we had wandered around the base of the wide mountain, making our way up slowly to get used to the altitude. The night would be a full-on charge up the rocky, gravelly remainder of the mountain. It was the most difficult part of the journey.

I knew the only way I was going to get my large body up the mountain was to power it through, and to do that I would need fuel. This wasn't bingeing, this was carbo-loading. We weren't particularly hungry; altitude is its own appetite suppressant. But eating now, before a day of fifteen hours of hiking, was imperative.

Every calorie would be gone by the following day.

Out of our group, I was the only one with a slight appetite. Having an appetite was the best possible scenario, because I could consume the energy I needed to get up the mountain. Still, I felt ashamed of it, as if I was supposed to be suffering and not eating. But I knew I needed energy. I needed enough food to get up the mountain, but not so much that I felt overstuffed or had to go to the bathroom. Let's just say it would be tricky to have to do number two that high, in a place so cold and exposed.

As we had gotten higher up the mountain, the food became less recognizable. The porters had to make dinners out of the leftovers, as it had been days since their supplies had been replenished. The food had to be nonperishable since there were no coolers or fridges along the way. That night, the porters made grilled cheese sandwiches in the shape of a triangle.

As I ate, Kenedy briefed us.

"We've decided that we need to leave at 11:00 PM," he told us. "You need more time."

Most climbing groups left at midnight.

Kenedy seemed tired of us—and now we would all get one less hour of sleep. We were, I imagined, exhausting for him.

But there was no getting around it. This was it, summit night (and day), which would mean twelve to fifteen hours of hiking to get to the top of the mountain and halfway down again. Whatever else we had accomplished up until that point, this was the day that really mattered. We were finally at the last stretch.

As I stepped out of the dining tent, I looked at the mountain. One last hurdle. I was sick of being uncomfortable. I missed my family and wanted to go home. Everything felt too heavy for me—including me. But first I'd have to get over this hump.

We were camping for the night near Kibo Hut, nothing more than a ramshackle cabin with cots. Some hikers stayed in the shelter, but I had read that it was impossible to sleep there because there were so many other anxious hikers around, trying to catch some shut-eye between their Diamox-fueled visits to the bathroom.

There was also a little ranger post with a store—nothing more than a few bottles of Coca-Cola and water in the window, but it was beautiful to me. I was so excited to hand someone money and get something back. It felt surreal, like civilization.

Other than for candy, I wasn't much of a shopper, but I felt positively giddy about purchasing a few bottles of clean water for the final six-mile stretch to the top. I rubbed my grimy fingers across them, then gulped down half a bottle before bed, which felt like magic as it unclogged my dusty throat.

Before I settled in, I popped by Stacey's tent to check on her. She hadn't taken off her boots. She was still in the clothes she had hiked in all day. She didn't even bother to sit up to talk with me. She put her arm over her forehead to block the sun penetrating her tent.

"I feel like shit. I have a really bad headache. It's pounding. It's in my neck." She let out a big sigh as she lifted her head to stretch her neck. She said she was too tired to take off her boots.

"If the headache goes away, I'll go up. If it doesn't go away . . ."

Neither one of us wanted to mention the alternative. She flopped hear head back down with a thud. "Ow."

Ultimately, it would be the guides' decision who went and how far up the mountain, but I hoped she wouldn't try to be a hero. As awful as it would be to make it to the last camp and not finish, her family didn't need another tragedy. I placed a water bottle and some of Sally and Tracey's extra energy gels in the alcove of her tent, as an offering. I sent a little wish into the sky, since I was among the stars, that she would recover enough to complete her mission.

CHAPTER 30

Unimpeded

DAY 4: MY MIND AT 15,580 FEET

"I know who I am and who I may be, if I choose."
—*Don Quixote de la Mancha.*

MY FATHER ONCE GAVE ME a Don Quixote statue: an iron figure without a base, it had burned during a fire at his house over Christmas break in 1985. It was one of the few visits we made to his home after the divorce. We had spent the holiday with my stepmother Helen and my father in Canada, didn't really get much love, attention, or gifts for that matter, and then came back to his home in Potsdam to find fire trucks around the smoldering structure.

The statue, which I plunked into a red Pacifica Mexican Cocoa candle so it could stay upright, reminded me that I too was on a quest. Every day I would go on a diet. Every night I ended in failure. On some level, I wished climbing Kilimanjaro would end that cycle.

It wasn't so wrong to help yourself while on a quest to do good. After all, I was hiking the mountain for myself, but also for AIDS orphans. Like Don Quixote, I was trying to slay giants and chase demons over the hill, except my windmills were the pounds on my body.

Being a plus-size person was its own kind of insanity. I was locked in a cycle of continually starting diets but never being able to seal the deal. It was an internal battle that consumed me from the moment I woke up. If only I could get it together, I often thought.

Sometimes I wondered if everyone thought I was mad for taking on Kilimanjaro.

If I was, I told myself that it wasn't so bad having something that I felt I must do. Other than the obvious must-do of shedding pounds, eating celery instead of cream puffs, the mountain was something I had to overcome. Sometimes, you have to listen to your heart to figure out where to go.

Crazy or not, fat or not, I didn't want to wake up one day filled with regret. I wanted to be a climber, a member of the club, even if I wasn't a good fit. Even if it meant becoming a crazy-ass person, hiking a mountain I had no place on.

The good thing about being on the mountain is you have all sorts of time to think. The bad thing about the mountain is that you have all sorts of time to think. I vowed that after this, I would go back home and everything would change.

But what if it didn't? What if everything remained exactly the same?

What if this was just a vacation, the same as any other? A mere blip in my routine. Like the six weeks I'd vow to lose weight before a wedding, a reunion, or any other gathering where I didn't want people to be whispering about my weight. I had this hurried sense of trying to get it right, of being on a deadline to get thin. I couldn't live like this anymore. It wasn't so much about the weight. The hardest part was the way I treated myself. The way I carried it all with me.

What if I could leave it here on the mountain?

Hikers typically work under the premise of leaving no trace, but I wanted to drop my metaphorical rubbish all over the mountain and let it float away in the wind. But maybe it wouldn't work that way. Maybe my weight would always be part of my story. That didn't mean I had to keep punishing myself for my past.

What if I could agree to just love myself? What if I could agree just this once—to love all that I am. What if I could move forward from here and be free? What if I could build a life that wasn't about diet or beauty, but about strength? Because underneath my layers, wasn't it true that my thighs most likely looked like a thoroughbred's? They'd have to, to carry all of me.

I needed not to feel less than others. I needed not to beat myself up with food. I need to nourish my soul, my body, my mind. Not with juice detoxes but with tasty raspberries. Walks filled with laughter. Lovemaking with my husband. Love in general.

Did I have it in me? Would I lose it when I wasn't forced to think about it, as I was on this mountain?

I needed some kind of epiphany—a sermon on the mount, with a tablet filled with life tenets to help me move forward, but not another diet book. I would have to create my own rules. I knew this for sure: the unhealthiest thing I could do was keep thinking this way about my body. I had to learn to be okay with who I was.

I fantasized about starting over and emptying out my cabinets the way I saw people do on reality diet shows. Kale. I could love kale. I would love kale.

I had to start whole as a complete person, as someone worthy of treating herself well. The sum of my parts—even the jiggly ones—made a greater whole.

I didn't want this journey, this final trip up the mountain, to have been for nothing. But all I could do was keep walking and see where the road took me. I had to see where I could go carrying all that I did, even if the hardest part was still ahead of me—even if it meant going back down the mountain again.

My biggest fear on this climb wasn't conquering the mountain, but conquering myself.

CHAPTER 31

Squished Lungs

DAY 4: KIBO HUT CAMP AND UPWARD, 15,580 FEET

As I BENT DOWN TO unlace my boots, I felt my lungs folding in half, and the world swirled around. I had to grip my tent top to find my balance, without ripping it from the ground.

I found my footing and tried again. I was dizzy. Not quite myself. I was living and breathing what little I could at 15,580 feet. Just doing so was exhausting. After a few minutes, I slipped inside my tent. I'd set it up to feel as much like home as possible, with my sleeping bag laid out and my duffle on the side where Chris would usually be. I opened up my bag and the stench of my stuff from the previous days on the trail overwhelmed me, even in the cold. I reached for the final Ziploc bag (the biggest, fullest one) for summit night. This one had my daughter's drawing of me on top of the mountain. It made me smile. I put it up to my face, and then quickly opened it to check its contents.

Inside were gloves, glove liners, a neck warmer, a hulky powder-blue plus-size parka, more long underwear (tops and bottoms), ski goggles in case it was windy on the top (with a crack on one side from one of my few attempts at skiing), a face warmer that made me look more like a bank robber than a hiker, and snow pants from Junonia because I have a 4X butt. I liked them because they had a drawstring so I didn't have to worry about using a bootlace if they were too loose after this week of hiking.

The gloves were my husband's. They were thick ski gloves, far too big for hiking a mountain, but when I sunk my hand inside, I felt a soft cushy happiness around my fingers, as if I was holding Chris's hand on the mountain.

I'd also brought gaiters to keep debris out of my beautiful boots; another fleece, which I'd been using as my pillow; sunglasses; extra Clif Bars; and of course my Camelbak and Nalgene bottle.

There's no telling what the weather would be on the summit. So you bundle up like the kid in *A Christmas Story* who couldn't put his arms down. As the sun comes up, you take off layer after layer.

My base layer was a moisture-wicking T-shirt that said, "Mind Over Mountain," which I'd worn the first time I summited. I loved it, even though it rolled up over my love handles. The rule of thumb for summit day was the less carried, the better. Essentials only: water, sunscreen, sunglasses, and a light snack—my stash of Clif Bars. We were about to traverse the most treacherous territory on Kilimanjaro.

The mountaintop, which was visible earlier in the hike from the gentle slope we had tread, was now out of sight. Our incline was straight up, like a roof pitch covered in sand. Every step moving forward would be a strenuous one. The weather had been great during our trek, but instead of it making me feel better, I worried that we'd used up our luck and would be walloped in the final day.

I tucked my hand-warmer packets inside my boots so they wouldn't freeze, then slipped into my sleeping bag wearing everything but my snow pants and jacket, so I could just pull those on when we got our 11:00 PM wake-up call.

On summit night you have to take care of your body, which was kind of ironic given what I'd done to my body over the years.

I knew if I could do this, I could do anything.

Oddly, despite yesterday's headache and occasional dizziness, I felt really good, even better than I had when I'd climbed to the peak the first time weighing 240 pounds. Maybe my good feelings were from having the knowledge of what was to come.

A friend of mine, who had also hiked Kilimanjaro three times, said the experience was a lot like childbirth. You forgot how hard it was until you were in it again. Especially when it came to summit night. I took off my socks, which were rank after so many days on the mountain. The smell overwhelmed my tent, but I didn't want to let any air out for fear of letting in the cold and snow that now frosted some of the rocks around the camp.

My tent felt like a pod, my private space for me to take care of what I needed to, without people looking at me or judging me. But it wasn't tall enough for all six feet of me, and that made preparing difficult.

I could hear Sally and Tracey in the neighboring tent, also hurrying to prepare for the last stretch.

I could also hear Tracey clearly struggling to breathe. I heard her digging through her summit-night bag, which contained all her gadgets, long underwear, long sleeves, long pants, clean underwear, and socks (a godsend). She also had her T-shirt from Team Z, her triathlon team, to remind her of her core group of friends who raised money for her.

I knew they meant to hoist it at the summit.

"Next time we unroll this, we'll be at the top," Sally said.

I didn't hear Tracey's response, just her labored breathing.

"I'm either going to be underdressed or overdressed so I'll shoot for overdressed, then leave room in my pack for the extra layers. I don't want to be underdressed because that would suck." It sounded like Sally was blabbering, trying to distract her friend.

We were instructed to leave our sleeping bags out. The porters would sleep in our tents while we were hiking to keep them safe and warm and to protect our stuff.

I peeked out of my tent and saw Sally pull out a Snickers.

"Aha, I have my secret weapon. Somebody told me it would work on summit day," Sally said. "It's a little melted, but it will do," she continued.

"You're funny," Tracey finally responded, pulling out her bag of energy gels and bars. "I'm having trouble thinking," I heard Tracey say. "I have all this food but do I have to take it with me? It makes me think that yesterday, when I was so tired, I could have eaten more and felt better," she said.

"Yeah, you don't want to leave anything behind, then wish you had it. That's so tricky," Sally said.

Tracey started singing the Beastie Boys song "Tricky."

Sally chimed in, "Tricky, tricky, tricky."

Tracey sorted through her bottle of pills, which I knew was a jumble of Diamox, Advil, Malarone, and more. They rattled as she moved them around.

They were going through their pre-summit checklist:

- *Take Diamox.*
- *Cut toenails.*
- *Double check boot laces.*
- *Sunglasses for the UV rays.*
- *Binoculars.*

"The thing about these bags is that you have to unpack everything to get what you want, and then you have to put it all back," Sally said.

Tracey said, "It's just arranging. Don't forget toilet paper."

But their list kept going on and on: hand warmers, flashlight, extra batteries, those are for my headlamp . . . more toilet paper.

"Yeah, shampoo, makeup remover, Oil of Olay . . . I don't think I need any of this," Sally said.

Tracey started laughing.

"Not one opportunity to use it at all," Sally said, holding the items up with a smirk. Tracey just giggled.

"Not even this, my facial cleanser," Sally said.

Tracey, trying to catch her breath, said, "I'm too tired to laugh . . . Stop."

I wanted to see them both succeed. They were so good to each other and for each other. I went to sleep hoping that I wasn't losing my comrade on the journey, Stacey. That I wasn't going to go it alone again.

After my things were in order, piled neatly at the foot of my tent, I decided to rest. I closed my eyes and surrendered.

It was dark. I was alone and afraid.

I wanted someone with me. I wanted someone to protect me. I wished my father was that person. I wished he could help me lace up my boots and pat me on the head for good luck on the journey ahead.

I put my hand on my heart as it accelerated in the low oxygen atmosphere and felt it beating as fast as if I were on the elliptical trainer.

I wondered what lurked within it. Was it scourging with plaque? Was it one step away from a heart attack?

My father had a history of heart disease. It had always been so awkward disclosing that to doctors when they collected family history. My family history was a box on a form. I had heart disease in my family—but the one with it wasn't around. Was I more at risk without him around? Or less?

I stretched my legs out and felt the true length of my body. I was as tall as my father. Six feet even. Our height was just enough to push us over the edge of six feet, something we both liked.

Below all this flesh was him. I carried him in my genetic map. What started as one cell from each parent became me. The femurs of my strong thighs, the fairness of my sunscreen-requiring face, the height of my being were all part of him. So perhaps he was there with me; he was cheering me on, even if he didn't know how to express it verbally.

CHAPTER 32

Losing It

DAY 5: SUMMIT ATTEMPT, 15,700 FEET

I COULD HEAR MY WAKE-UP call before it arrived, although the guides moved as softly as they could, trying to be respectful of the other campers. But there was no escaping the rustle of their getting breakfast ready for the four of us, Kenedy, and Michael.

In the dark, just outside my tent, I heard the crunch, crunch, crunch of footsteps, and saw a bouncing headlight.

"Mama Kubwa," Michael said. "It's time."

"I'm up. I'm up," I said, tapping to the left of my sleeping bag to find my headlamp. I had put it in my sleeping bag so the batteries wouldn't die in the cold. I reached down to find the elastic band, looped it around my fingers, and pulled it up over my head.

I hadn't really slept, but whatever rest I'd gotten would have to be enough now.

I sat up at a right angle and shone the light on my stuff at the edge of my tent, exposing my back to the cold. I reached over to grab fleece after fleece to cover up, five layers in all. I held the gaiters I had rented; they didn't fit around my calves. I needed them to keep tiny stones from the scree surface of the summit attempt out of my boots. They were especially important on the way down when the icy surface melts in the sunlight and frees the little rocks.

I could hear Stacey chatting with Michael outside, so I pulled on my jacket and fumbled out of my tent, making my way over tent strings to see them.

"Are you wearing two mid-weight hiker socks together or a liner and a big one?" she asked when I poked my head in her tent.

Her question caught me by surprise. I had been expecting her to tell me she was ready to go back down the mountain, but here she was, awake and seemingly chipper about the twenty-mile trek ahead.

"A liner and a big one," I said, feeling the cushy softness around my toes.

She handed me duct tape to cover my Camelbak water tube with plumbers' insulation—a trick to keep it from freezing. As I gave her a once-over, I couldn't help thinking she looked so good it was almost as if she was faking earlier.

She showed me her empty water bottle. "I must have peed six times," she said.

"Great," I said, with pride that she was taking care of herself.

"I ate all the snacks that Tracey and Sally left for me," Stacey said.

"We wanted to make sure you had enough to eat," I said. "I'm so glad you look better. I was worried about you," I admitted.

"Yeah, I didn't think I was going to be able to do this," she said, quickly shifting back to the business at hand. "I have about twenty layers on."

"You look fabulous," I said.

"I feel really hot. No really, it's super-warm," Stacey said. "I'm not sure I can get the Camelbak out of my backpack if I have all this stuff on."

"If the wind kicks up, you'll need that stuff. If you don't, you can just take it off," I said.

"I'm nervous about having to pee with all this stuff on," Stacey said.

"You'll be okay," I said. "Do the best you can to go before we get out there."

I could feel I was mothering again, so I backed out of her tent before I said another word.

Outside, I looked up at the crescent moon. The blanket of stars was not just above me, but all around, even below me.

My headlamp shone a straight line to my tent. I could see in front of me but I felt a little wobbly. I put on my gaiters to see what I could do about them, grabbed an empty water bottle, and headed to the mess tent. When I got there, Michael looked down at the gaiters hanging off my ankles.

"Duct tape?" he said.

"I think that's our best bet," I replied.

He got down on his knees and wrapped the rolls of silver tape around the forest-green gaiters, securing them to my legs. All my layers plus my Camelbak tube made me feel like a robot as I moved over to my bucket to take my seat.

This morning, the dining tent was set up like a continental breakfast. The chef had been working to boil our water, but at that altitude, he couldn't get it up to the right temperature to make oatmeal. Still, it sat steaming on the table, then turned cold almost as soon as we spooned it out.

It felt unnatural eating at ten o'clock at night, but I tried, and took a couple of biscuits, just in case.

"Okay, everyone. It's time," Kenedy said.

We lined up behind Michael, the moon lighting our way. As we waited, we checked zippers, secured our balaclavas around our faces, and adjusted turtlenecks. We looked like miners with our headlamps peering out into the darkness.

The only thing left to do was walk.

CHAPTER 33

Deep Dark

DAY 5: SUMMIT DAY, ABOUT 16,000 FEET

WALKING ON A MOUNTAIN IN the dark was daunting. We had to trust our guides. We had to trust ourselves.

The dark removed all other distractions. It was too cold to look down at gadgets. There was nothing to see except the spotlight of our headlamps illuminating the gravelly scree below our feet.

Walking on the scree without losing my footing took tremendous focus. Each of us had to lean into the hill, hoping the ground would support us and keep us moving in the right direction. Lean back and you'd end up right where you'd started, at the bottom of the mountain.

I tried to empty my mind, to let myself be enveloped by the night, to live in that quiet space while the rest of the world was asleep, dreaming, snug and safe in their beds.

There was no letting your thoughts drift over the horizon, no looking back to where you had been. Your headlamp illuminated only where you needed to go next—the few steps right in front of you.

For once, our group was in lockstep, like a train to the top. The only sounds were our feet tramping on the gravel. If I just kept moving,

I knew I could keep this up. I was on the slowest train in the world, but still I was grinding along.

Suddenly, taking another step felt painfully hard. Heat radiated from my chest. I tried to shake off the burning discomfort, but the weight of it made me feel like I was about to vomit up my breakfast.

But it just wouldn't come.

This nausea had nothing to do with eating greasy food or overindulging. We were taking our bodies to the limit, at an altitude that would have been tough for anyone, not just two fat girls like Stacey and me.

Our bodies were speaking to us. In the dark, in the cold, with nothing else to distract us, we had to listen. The burning feeling was heartburn as our stomachs and every other organ reeled in the high-altitude conditions.

An hour into the hike, we could see glimmers of other hikers below us, making their way up the mountain. With each step, their headlamps got brighter. They had all left at midnight and were gaining on us.

Walking up the trail through the stars had been exciting for the first hour. Maybe even the second hour. By the third hour, the camp was out of sight and we were feeling lost—floating in space. It wasn't fun anymore, just a long mountain slog. Even the guides, who had been singing as we walked, fell mostly silent.

I wondered if I was crazy, putting my life in the hands of people who had insulted me, doubted me. But I had to have faith they were taking me in the right direction. I had to trust them. And myself. If I stopped, I knew I wouldn't be able to start again.

My breathing was heavy, like an ocean tide. Inhaling was the rolling to shore, exhaling was the crashing on the sand. It felt as if breathing and walking were my body's only jobs.

In my mind, I counted the milestones we'd pass before the summit: Williams Point, Jamaica Rocks, and Gilman's Point.

These were my benchmarks. Things I could look forward to, like scenes in a movie, except I couldn't fast-forward. With three more hours to go before Gilman's Point, it started to seem as if I would again end in failure.

Tracey had fallen behind. Spending the night at 15,580 feet was too much. Even though she started the day with her game face on, she struggled from the start.

I later learned she had taken off her gloves to reach for her water, but it was frozen. She tried to swig her cloudy reserve bottle, and then fumbled to put her gloves back on. I could see her struggling with her glove liners, trying to pull them up, every second in the cold making it more difficult for her to move her hands. She reached into her pocket for her hand warmers, but lost her balance.

I saw her sit down, right on the trail, gasping in panic.

She looked down at her heart-rate monitor. Her breath came in ever quickening gasps, but her pulse was slowing. It was down to eighty. Her pulse should have been quickening in the high altitude.

"I can't. I can't breathe," she said, looking up at Kenedy from the rock.

He ushered us ahead, and our group continued to advance. Tracey could only watch as she slowly became detached, like a caboose left on the rails. We were at 17,400 feet.

She told us later that Kenedy had quietly told her, "It is time to go down."

"I know," she'd told him and started to cry.

She handed Kenedy her Team Z flag to give to Sally and disappeared down into the darkness with one of the porters.

Knowing that Tracey had to go back down gave me no satisfaction, even though she had been critical of me. Seeing people heading down the mountain instead of up, arm in arm with a porter, a sullen look on their faces, was disappointing. The reality was anyone could have to turn around. It could still happen to me. I wanted Tracey to see me at the top. I wanted to see her at the top, too.

KENEDY HAD TO WALK DOUBLE-TIME, something only an experienced, acclimatized mountain man could do, to catch up with our group before our headlamps vanished on the horizon. It was the first time I had seen him out of breath.

Then he had to tell Sally that her best friend had gone down and wouldn't make it to the summit.

"She couldn't breathe and decided she needed to stop and turn back. We can't let her go up because she is going to miss the oxygen," he told Sally. "She is with Richard, the porter who came with us."

It suddenly became clear that Richard was with us as someone to shepherd hikers in trouble back down the mountain.

"It's hard for me to imagine going up this mountain without Tracey. She's . . ." Sally stopped, wracked by sobs, which I knew would only make it difficult for her to breathe too ". . . my best friend. I don't know what to do."

I could see Kenedy trying to negotiate, trying to manage Sally's emotions while getting us all to the top of the mountain. Every moment we stopped to talk in the freezing temperatures hindered our ability to go on.

"Don't think about her. Don't think about her. She's okay, she's fine. Just try to go up," Kenedy said.

But Sally still sobbed. "We'd promised that if one of us goes down, the other would go up. But it's hard," Sally said.

"Don't think about her. If you feel good, let's go up," Kenedy urged again, pointing out the Team Z flag. "Let's go up, please. Don't think about her. She's fine. She's fine. Believe me, please."

Sally still sobbed, the headlamp illuminating the tears forming then freezing on her cheeks like little crystals. She took a deep breath, but I could see her slipping, her will to move forward waning.

"Here, we'll get you through it. Come here, Sally, we'll get you there," I said, reaching out my hand.

But the news of Tracey going down had shattered the group's confidence. As much as I tried to muster up renewed optimism, still trying to be the leader, the possibility of us all turning back was real. I couldn't stop myself from thinking Tracey was already on her way down and she was way stronger than I was.

"I should go down, too. I can't just leave her," Sally sniveled.

"Do it for her," Kenedy implored. "Do it for her."

"Okay, I will do it for her," Sally said. Her face was red from crying and exhaustion.

"We can do this," I said, but now that Tracey was gone, I wasn't sure.

I KNEW FROM EXPERIENCE HOW hard it was to turn around, to end at the bottom, only to start all over again, to be so deep into something, and have your body put on the brakes.

Hiking Kilimanjaro requires a constant balance between what your mind and body are saying to you. The mind gives up a lot sooner than the body, making it tough to know if you're really in trouble or if you're just making excuses, calling it quits before you've reached your full potential.

Are you giving up on yourself or is your body doing it for you?

If you take one more step, will you be successful or will you be putting yourself in grave danger?

The guides are trained to look for major signs of trouble: stumbling while walking, talking gibberish, and shortness of breath while just standing. But only we could know for sure if we were truly hurting.

We were far from any hospital, the only saving grace being some supplemental oxygen and hope the guides were indeed CPR certified.

As much as I was comforting Sally, I knew I had to comfort myself.

This is not where my story ends, I thought. But I couldn't help wondering if my resentment of Tracey had somehow gotten in the way of her success.

Did I make it happen? Was it my fault? Maybe I'd be next?

This I cannot change. I am here. I am on the mountain, and I have to haul my ass up to the summit. So I'd better dig in.

That thought sustained me for the next hour. I let this reminder turn over in my brain as I just walked.

I COULDN'T DRINK. THE WATER tube of my Camelbak was frozen solid. I pursed my chapped lips but try as I might to suck the water out, it wouldn't budge. I chomped down on the nozzle and my teeth immediately stung from the cold. I took my gloves off to try to maneuver the nozzle into a place free from ice. My hands started to freeze. I made fists inside Chris's gloves, thinking of him, hoping each one would warm the other.

When I held up my white fingers to my headlamp, I felt like I was turning into a corpse. Quickly, I pulled up my glove liners and then thrust my hands back into my mittens. It didn't matter. I couldn't feel the tips of my fingers. Panicked, I imagined coming home with my hands permanently damaged: a writer, unable to write. All for this stupid mountain. Negative thoughts swirled around my head, tugging me down into darkness.

"I don't remember this being so hard," I said, throwing my hiking poles down on the ground. "This sucks. This was the worst idea ever to come back here."

This tantrum didn't sit well with the two remaining hikers in my group. I had organized our little expedition, and I was unraveling.

Stacey just said, "Come on, Kara. Get it together." I watched her mumble something to Sally, probably about me, and huff away, showing how displeased she was.

I couldn't think clearly. I couldn't even see them clearly. With their headlamps on, it was like staring down oncoming traffic.

"It's okay," Sally said, comforting me this time. "You can do it. Just remember: pole, pole. Slowly, slowly."

Easy for her to say, I thought, looking over at her perky red parka and blond hair, which still looked neat under her hat despite five days without a shower. The taut little newscaster didn't have to carry around the weight of a 120-pound person on her back. Sally had been my friend for years but that night I wanted to strangle her for roping me into this trek. Or was it I who roped her into it? The details were getting fuzzy. I was angry with everyone.

CHAPTER 34

Frozen

DAY 5: BEFORE DAWN, 17,000 FEET

I WAS JUST A FEW hours from the summit, and I was beginning to think I had made a huge mistake. I was smelly, sweaty, exhausted, and struggling to breathe.

Stacey trudged along in front of me, digging her hiking poles into the ground. She probably wanted to dig them into me but didn't want to waste any energy.

"Come on, Kara," she practically growled at me from behind her black balaclava. Her normally engaging brown eyes looked down at the ground, as if she didn't want to see me struggling, to get the image out of her head so she could continue.

I could barely bend down to pick up my poles. My quads burned, my calves shrieked, my pants sank down and exposed the small of my large back.

I hated that I had put myself in such a terrible position—too fat to hike the mountain. Too fat for anything.

It was impossible to see the jagged ridge, Gilman's Point, in front of us against the night sky. It was a mystery as to where it really was. The only clue was to look for where the stars stopped, but most times, our heads were down, sizing up the contours of the uneven ground below.

Before the trip, Sally and Tracey had vowed to raise $19,343—$1 per foot of the mountain—if I came along. How could I say no?

But what I really should have said no to were pie, cupcakes, cookies, and chips.

I should have said no to skipping workouts.

I should have said no to mindlessly tinkering on Facebook instead of facing my weight demons.

I knew that with my extra pounds, the summit could very well be out of reach for me.

It took everything I had to move my feet, one in front of the other, always sliding back, as if I were lifting shackles and chains. I could hear my mother's voice in my head: "I wish I could be absolutely certain that you'd come back." Me, too. I felt a searing pain in my back, beyond the burden of my girth. I couldn't blame my daypack; it was nearly empty, but it felt too heavy to bear. It was cold enough to freeze my water bottle, but I had already shed my clunky blue parka and given it to our head guide Kenedy to carry. I couldn't bear the extra weight. I hated asking for help, but I needed him and surrendered the parka, hoping it would be enough to get me through.

A wave of nausea surged through me. I put my hand on a rock and lunged forward. I wanted to vomit, but I had nothing left inside me.

Now, at about 17,000 feet, it didn't matter who I was or what I weighed. The mountain didn't care about any of that.

CHAPTER 35

Dark Times

DAY 5: WILLIAMS POINT, 16,404 FEET

THE ACRID BODY ODOR COULDN'T have been his—the family friend who had sexually assaulted me—but in my head, I thought it was. It was the same smell of teenage sweat, the same smell that overwhelmed me when he had climbed on top of me on my twelfth birthday. I felt as if my predator were about to sneak up behind me and do it again.

I was at 16,404 feet, climbing higher with each step, yet I couldn't escape the smell. Maybe it was coming from me? Maybe it was coming from the guides? Maybe it was coming from my increasingly addled mind?

Here I was, struggling to breathe, to move forward, yet I was stuck in the putrid stench of the past.

My body had used up the energy from breakfast—toast and oatmeal that was barely palatable in the thin air. Seeing that we were struggling, Kenedy found us a spot to rest for a few minutes at Williams Point—a glorified outcropping of rocks, and the second milestone to the summit—but we couldn't pause for long. It was minus-ten degrees. I reached for a Clif Bar, but it was frozen solid. I threw it down in disgust. "I can't even eat."

When I needed food—and comfort—the most, it wasn't there for me. The memory made it harder to keep climbing. The fact that it was there troubled me. I wanted to be past it but the only way to get over being stuck with it there at Williams Point was to keep climbing.

"I feel awful but I'm not stopping," I said to Sally and Stacey. I was the leader of this expedition, and I needed to continue. I had gotten myself on the mountain. I was going to have to get myself off it.

I had mutilated myself with food year after year. Now I had to carry the results with me day in and day out.

I wanted to blame everyone and everything else. My gloves were too thin. My boots were too heavy. With each step I took, my feet dug deeper into the scree, making it more difficult to move. I could see that my bitching and moaning were holding up the group. I had a choice: stand still or keep going. Going back was not an option.

This is where most of my efforts to lose weight stopped. When it got tough. When I started to feel scared of failure.

In many ways, my weight served me. Because of my unusual shape—small on top with size twenty-eight pants—people remembered me. They remembered my name. They remembered my story. I was the fat girl who hiked mountains. After growing up with divorced parents who didn't notice me, I got a lot of attention for being big.

Here in the dark, I couldn't escape this thought: I made myself a monster.

I did this.

CHAPTER 36

Stripping

DAY 5: JAMAICA ROCKS, 17,000 FEET—ABOUT 5:00 AM

THE TRAIL ON THE WOBBLY Jamaica Rocks section of the mountain was like petrified kitty litter mixed with jagged volcanic rock. But it felt like my feet were trapped in Jell-O or quicksand. One misstep and I could fall and smash my skull on a rock, my brains dripping off the sides of the narrow path. That was if cerebral edema from the high altitude or the subfreezing temperatures didn't get me first.

We'd been hiking for six hours and the hardest part was ahead of us. We had another hour to Gilman's Point. I was already shot. Each moment that I moved made me desperate to rest.

The trouble with facing your demons on the mountain is that you still have to get down safely without the aid of those excuses. It would be hard work living without this story I had blanketed myself with for so many years. How would I not get lost on the way down?

I started to shiver with this thought. Despite the cold, I started to undress. I handed my backpack to Kenedy. I stripped off layer after layer of clothing to feel lighter. Just as I had done on my weekly visits to Weight Watchers, hoping for a lower number on the scale.

I gave my parka and fleece to Michael. Each ounce made a difference and helped me feel stronger. I needed their help. I couldn't do this alone.

AN HOUR LATER, I COULD see Sally ahead in the distance approaching the outcropping of rocks, the cove that held the Gilman's Point sign. Our endpoint.

I could hear another climber over the rocks, already there, encouraging her. "A few more steps and you're golden."

"*Asante sana*. Thank you. Thank you," Sally called back. "I wanted to quit so many times but I kept saying that I wanted to do it for both of us." She grabbed for the Gilman's Point sign and disappeared into the nest of rocks.

I wanted to be happy for her. But I couldn't. At my speed, it could take me at least thirty minutes to get to where she was, although the end was in sight.

My body shook from exhaustion. I just didn't know if I had it in me anymore.

We'd been hiking all night; now the sun was well on its way into the sky. I needed to get on up the mountain before the altitude stopped me.

"I'm never doing this again," Stacey said. "I can't wait to go home."

"Um-hm," was all I could reply.

A few steps more and I could see them—what so few people have set eyes upon—the disappearing glaciers of Kilimanjaro.

"I see glaciers. That's pretty amazing. They're beautiful. Kind of makes it worth the trip," I called up to Sally, partially to let her know that I was still breathing. Then added, "This is way harder than I remember. Way harder."

Stacey, seeing Sally's accomplishment, seemed to double-time her way to the top, leaving me hunched over and wanting to hurl.

"I just need to catch my breath," Stacey said, up above near the ridge, where I could hear the rounds of congratulations brewing. "That was tough."

Kenedy directed me to keep walking, the same way I directed my daughter to put her shoes on.

"Just try to make it to the summit," he said.

"I feel like I'm going to throw up. I could really use some food. I feel like that would help quell my stomach. I'm exhausted. I am just so exhausted," I said. "I just want to get to Gilman's and be done."

I waited and tried to summon the strength to continue.

"Three minutes. Three minutes. I can do anything for three minutes," I said. I held my head for a second, looking down at the gray rock below. Thousands upon thousands of boulders and rocks at my feet. Each one on top of the next one formed an endless pile for me to stand on, reaching up to my feet, supporting me.

The first sight of the sun was just a glimmer, a ray above the clouds. Little by little, it revealed itself until the entire sky above the gray, wavy clouds was orange.

At this elevation, climbing Kilimanjaro became a moving meditation, and I revisited my mantra from my spin-class instructor: Strong. Steady. Smooth.

I let the words roll over me. I tried to say them out loud but I didn't have the breath.

Strong. Steady. Smooth. Strong. Steady. Smooth. Strong. Steady. Smooth.

We were supposed to arrive at Gilman's Point by sunrise. But as the horizon below me began to glow, I knew I was late. But I couldn't rush. I'd take a few steps, then rest. I was moving, as my father used to say, "like molasses in January."

That I was. But I kept going. As much as I detested how my father left me, he was still in me. I could take the best of him, his strength and stubbornness, and use it for my own good. The people in our lives are gifts.

My feet felt stuck in cement blocks. But I kept looking up, toward the summit, and thought, I'm a tough motherfucker, and proud of it. Gilman's Point seemed like an oasis, something that we'd been approaching but would never reach. For hours, other groups had passed us by. Now that the sun was on its way up, I could see everyone celebrating at the top.

Michael stayed with me. He paused when I needed to pause but told me to keep on.

"Pole, pole, Mama Kubwa," he said. "Slowly, slowly."

I looked down at my feet, willing them to move.

Again and again, I went through this agonizing process: just one step.

Then I heard Kenedy's voice. "Mama Kubwa made it."

CHAPTER 37

Kiss the Sign

DAY 5: GILMAN'S POINT, 18,638 FEET—MORNING, WAY BEYOND SUNRISE

I GRABBED THE WOOD OF the crooked Gilman's Point sign and let it help me on the final step to the lookout.

"I'm going to kiss this sign," I said.

In that moment of reaching the summit, I was out of breath and wanted to cry. I looked above me and tried to control my tears, but there I was, clutching the sign.

"We're here," I said. "We're here."

"Mama Kubwa made it, you guys. Mama Kubwa made it," Kenedy said, as if he had never doubted it for a minute.

At 18,638 feet, I was standing on the roof of Africa, a point so high nothing could touch me. I looked out and could see and believe I was there. I had made it.

The ridges of Mawenzi were painted brightly by the sun. All of Africa was spread out below us, a vast, curved horizon.

Finally, I wasn't moving. I was still. I could enjoy the view and the accomplishment and each breath of air.

I leaned into the rocks, wanting to melt into them, as if there were a bench for me carved into them. I wanted to take a nap.

These were signs of altitude sickness. I was exhausted as I pushed my back into the rocks that made up Gilman's Point. It was the first comfortable seat I'd found since I started this journey.

"I need something to eat," I said, realizing I had been hiking for six hours without a snack. "I'm so hungry," and for once, I was. It was a true hunger—a feeling of being empty. A purity, a need.

Stacey handed me a Clif Bar, but I kept forgetting I had it in my hand.

My spirit soared above the peaks, but my body needed sustenance. I was thirsty. I lapped up water, half frozen like a Slurpee, from my wide-mouth bottle. It hadn't occurred to me to drink from it earlier. I didn't have the energy on the trail.

"I'm so grateful," I bellowed in a weepy diatribe. "Grateful for all the people who supported me along the way; from my trainer to my guides, everyone was there for me. Every step through the darkness led to this."

I dove into a hug with Sally, Stacey, Kenedy, and Michael. This was a Gatorade-dumping-over-the-head moment and I was glad to have their arms to hold me up.

CHAPTER 38

Asante

DAY 5: GILMAN'S POINT TO HOROMBO HUTS, 18,815 TO 12,204 FEET

GETTING TO THE TOP OF the mountain wasn't enough. Now I had to go all the way down. I needed to find the strength to get there. I needed to make the mountain my own.

But first, Stacey had something to do. She pulled a vial out of her pocket and walked to the rim. She inhaled deeply, her eyes bubbling over.

With trembling hands, Stacey removed her glove and uncapped the silver vial. Looking toward the crater, she set her mother's ashes free. The cloud of ash was gray at first, then blended into the landscape—the vast crater of the mountain and the majestic white glaciers under a brightening blue sky.

Stacey started to cry.

I walked up behind her and she turned to look at me. "Are you ready?"

We hugged, after the ashes had settled on the mountain. I could see her dad's dog tags around her neck. They clinked against me as Stacey sobbed.

Her inhales were short as she was gasping for oxygen.

Our time at Gilman's Point was short. Each moment we stayed there, we felt as if we were dying, losing our breath. Despite the physical discomfort, here on top of Mount Kilimanjaro, I felt as if I could start to let go.

I made it. I made it. I made it.

Nothing else in the world mattered. I cried for all I had done to get up the mountain—for facing my fear and walking through it.

I cried because my quad muscles felt shredded, my calves felt like boulders, and now we needed to go down and fast.

We couldn't gingerly sidestep down the slope; the only way down was to scree run.

Looking down, it was hard to believe that I had made it up something so long, so steep. If I had dropped my water bottle, it might roll all the way back to camp.

Scree running meant launching ourselves forward, as if jumping into the snow, and running down the pebbles and loose rocks of the mountainside.

Sally had hurried down with another group to reunite with and check on Tracey. Stacey and I held on to our guides as we began our descent. She was with Kenedy. I was with Michael. It was kind of fun.

We made it down at breakneck speed, around the jagged rocks and zigzag trails that brought us so high, back down to Kibo Hut for a break and to meet Tracey before heading down the Marangu Route. What had taken us three days to go up took us six hours to go down.

Letting myself go at the top of this mountain, I worried I would tumble and roll like a menacing boulder down the slope. My biceps and shoulders tightened as I thrust my hiking poles into the ground, trying to brace my weight and protect my knees.

Every step down in altitude made us stronger. We could finally breathe. The thrill of our accomplishment and the extra oxygen gave us an extra adrenaline surge down the mountain. Plus, going downhill is just less taxing. My hiking poles buffered my knees as I bounced down the mountain.

But word of my success made it down to Kibo Hut Camp before

I did. Every porter on their way up and down expressed some kind of congratulations. "Wow, I heard about you," one porter said, as he headed up to resupply his team. "Amazing."

Part of me wanted to say, "In your face," to the porters who doubted me, except I was kind of surprised myself. So when each one stopped me to say, "Well done, Mama Kubwa," I stopped to take it in and say, "Thank you."

Too tired to take off my boots, I dove into my tent. I sat up only to pour water into my throat. I remembered the biscuits for a moment but just closed my eyes instead.

AFTER A TWO-HOUR NAP, I checked in with the porters, who were gathered and ready to go. Michael and Kenedy looked exhausted. I told them about all the comments and compliments down the mountain.

"Many people say they can't believe she made it. But she made it. Congratulations. It was good, Mama," Michael said.

It was the first time he didn't say *kubwa*. I was just Mama.

"Nobody believes this because you are very fat. To me, a woman or man who is very fat normally can't do Kilimanjaro . . . it is hard work but you did it," said Kenedy. "It was a surprise for anyone who saw you passing on the road."

I felt like I had earned my keep. I belonged no matter what anyone thought of me.

Almost on autopilot, my legs moved me down the mountain, letting the lactic acid rinse out. With each breath of oxygen, I felt stronger, almost giddy. Although the insides of my thighs were raw and the blister on my foot burned, it didn't matter. I was heading home.

WE CAMPED AT HOROMBO HUTS for the night, our last dinner on the mountain.

Tracey shared her story, still trying to calculate what had gone wrong and how she could have improved it. She talked about how everything was at an angle on the mountain slope and she could never quite get her bearings, but at a lower altitude she was recovering. She was feeling better. Tracey shared how horrible she had felt when she turned back.

She had no intention of returning to the mountain.

Neither did I. I was complete—and full. Except for one thing.

I called my family.

"I made it to the top. I'm okay," I said. I was okay.

It was just a voicemail. It was Anna's bedtime, and I knew this was an all-hands-on deck endeavor with bath, stories, and soothing. I wanted to be with her. I wanted to hear their voices, their cheers. But for now, it would have to come from within me.

THERE IS A TRADITION AMONG Kilimanjaro trekkers to thank your porters with a ceremony. They sing a song, a celebration of how far you've come, and line up like a chorus.

> *Leader: Kilimanjaro*
> *Chorus: Kilimanjaro, mlima mrefu sana*
> *Leader: Na Mawenzi*
> *Chorus: Na Mawenzi, Na Mawenzi . . . Na Mawenzi,*
> *   Na Mawenzi mlima mrefu sana*
> *Leader: Ewe Nyoka*
> *Chorus: Ewe Nyoka, Ewe Nyoka . . . Ewe Nyoka, Ewe Nyoka*
> *   mbona wanizunguka*
> *Leader: Wanizunguka*
> *Chorus: Wanizunguka, Wanizunguka . . . Wanizunguka,*
> *   Wanizunguka wataka kunila nyama*

The song is about Kilimanjaro, the really tall mountain. Then it goes a little off topic. The last bit means: "You snake, why are you circling me? You're circling me because you want to eat me."

I never put too much significance on the meaning: just a fun little ditty before we handed out tips (because by the end of the journey, you're ready to sign over the deed of your home to these guys). But hearing it one last time, I had to wonder what this was all about. I started to think about it in the context of my struggle with food. It had been eating me alive, so consuming that I didn't know how to enjoy, to live, to be present.

"We want so much to thank you for all that you've done this week. You've helped us . . . conquer everything . . . carrying our bags . . . so we thank you so very, very much," I said to the porters.

Despite their earlier comments and doubts, I thanked them. For that, I was a stronger person.

But we still had one more day of going down. A half marathon—13.1 miles—to the bottom of the mountain.

Fortunately, I was carrying a lot less baggage.

CHAPTER 39

Booted

DAY 6: MARANGU GATE, 5,413 FEET

As WE HEADED AWAY FROM camp, I looked up to see the silhouette of the mountain. I was taking firm steps away from it, to new adventures, new experiences.

Even though every motion down the mountain meant more glorious oxygen filling our lungs, each step hurt.

I removed my right boot and sock to find that my big toe was red, raw, and ready to explode. My Band-Aids were in my backpack, miles down the trail. Oh yes, and so was my water. Michael and Kenedy headed down the mountain to make sure our bus was ready when we got there.

My tongue felt like a pumice stone. Squeezing my foot back into my boot was the last thing I wanted to do, but we had a lot more ground to cover. It takes five and a half days to hike up Kilimanjaro. On the way down, the same distance is covered in a day and a half.

Ed Viesturs, a mountaineering legend who conquered the world's fourteen highest peaks, has an unwavering policy: "Reaching the summit is optional. Getting down is mandatory."

In fact, you're more likely to die or get injured on the way down a mountain than on the way up. Being tired, sloppy, and just wanting the climb to be over can lead to some serious injuries or missteps.

Case in point: me. On the way down Africa's highest peak, I was clumsily dragging myself down the mountain, tripping over rocks as I sloughed my feet through the dust. I hardly noticed the vegetation returning around me, first the bushes, then the trees. Even though I was concentrating on getting down the mountain, I was returning to life.

Without the adrenaline from the quest to get to the peak, each step felt like an electric bolt up my right leg. My toes jammed into the front of my boot. I knew I would pay the price in toenails, perhaps even losing one on the trail itself.

A friend had once given me the solid advice to trim your toenails before taking on a big hike. Otherwise, they jam into the top of your boots. But this trek was too much for even the most perfectly pedicured feet. Just touching the toenail caused searing pain. I could feel a blister building below the nail itself and all around the nail bed. I would have gnawed it off to release the pressure if I could, except I couldn't lift my toe to my mouth.

My fellow hikers were plowing down the mountain, envisioning hot showers and cold beers. I wanted to keep up with them, but my boots had become my enemy. I had to squeeze them back on and keep going.

This pair—Asolo 520s—had been my hiking companions over the years. I bought them for my first Kilimanjaro hike. I remember feeling the strong, smooth leather and hard rubber soles, thinking I would never be able to lift them off the ground. They weighed two pounds each. Even heftier was the price tag: $289.

Now, I just wanted to be rid of them. I even envisioned ceremoniously setting them on fire at the hotel to celebrate their three treks up Mount Kilimanjaro, not to mention all the hiking in between. Our assistant guide, Michael, had been wearing Skechers throughout the trek. While they are fine casual shoes, they had no place on the mountain. There was no tread, or ankle support, or warmth.

One of the warnings many Kilimanjaro guidebooks give is to make sure that each member of the crew has proper footwear. But proper footwear can be loosely defined. I've seen some porters in other expeditions wearing flip-flops, others in dress shoes, while carrying thirty-five pounds of hikers' belongings on their head.

If the boots fit Michael, I would give them to him. That way they could stay on Kilimanjaro forever, where they belonged. Not that I didn't want to hike anymore, but three times up Kilimanjaro was enough. If I was going to be free of my issues, this weight, I needed to start heading in a different direction.

Just as with the boots, I could decide to let go of the things that no longer served me.

AT THE BASE OF THE mountain, we saw our things scattered on the lawn, ready to be loaded on the bus.

I took off my boots and handed them to Michael. I slipped my feet into my hard-sole slippers, hoping the blister brewing behind my big toenail wouldn't pop. Then I hobbled onto the bus.

CHAPTER 40

Downtime

NGORONGORO CRATER

Our trip included four days of fun before departure. We would spend a few days on safari and then jet off to Zanzibar, one of the Spice Islands off the coast of Tanzania, to rest our legs. There were many Tusker beers also involved in our recovery, as we sipped and savored our accomplishment before trekking across the hotel lobby for a shower.

At the hotel before the safari, Stacey and I shared a room. She called dibs on the shower. After a moment, I heard a shriek, "What the fuck? What the fuck?"

The shower was just a dribble of lukewarm water.

We had been dreaming of a shower for days, and now it wasn't going to be the Irish Spring moment we were waiting for. My heart sank, but it still felt wonderful to have a roof over our heads, even if our beds had to be covered in mosquito nets. What little warm water we had would be used by Stacey's attempt to get clean.

I stood with freezing water dripping over me, dirt swimming down to the drain, as I soaped up as many times as I could stand. I had hurried too much to get clean, as the white towel was brown by the time I had finished drying off.

I had hoped to return four (or more) sizes smaller. Of course, that was a ridiculous thing to want, but I couldn't help but think of Kilimanjaro as a weight-loss effort. My clothes were hanging on me. My muscles felt taut, which made me want to eat something healthy. I wanted to take care of this body, the one that was feeling strong and free.

We picked from a buffet. I had a glass of wine and some seafood. My plate felt balanced—and nothing more. No helpings of guilt. No overindulgence. It was exactly what I needed. I smiled with delight since I was the one in control of the serving spoons. It wasn't a Lean Cuisine or a full-out postclimb treat. It was just food and it was delicious.

THE NEXT DAY WE HEADED into the Ngorongoro Crater, a large, flat caldera, home to 25,000 animals—from flamingos to hippos. The roads were a jumble of rocky zigzags, and as we bumped along, I flopped and flailed, my muscles too weak to hold me steady. We paid for the safari as an add-on to the vacation. It was our treat, our reward, for working so hard.

Our safari drivers spent the day in search of the big five—rhinoceroses, lions, leopards, elephants, and buffalo—the prizes of safari watching. After hours of popping our heads out of the Land Rover and snapping photos, we finally spotted an elephant, and my heart soared. He was a beautiful gray being, with tusks curving up to the sky. I watched him making his way across the plain, slow and steady.

I know how you feel, I thought.

Mount Kilimanjaro was now just part of the background. It was behind me. I didn't have to keep climbing over and over again. I didn't have to lose weight to be worthy of being on top of the mountain. I had the strength within me all along. I was whole and unbroken. I did have it together.

I'd spent my life covering myself over, pound by pound. Now, pound by pound, I wanted to uncover what had been eating away at me all those years. Like a mountain slog, it would be a long, grueling process. I was the one who had to do it, but I didn't have to be on Kilimanjaro to do it.

I wanted to stop running away and be grateful for what I already had—my husband, my beautiful daughter—instead of wishing my life, my past, was different. For me, the key to stop comfort eating is to remind myself that, despite my past, I'm not empty.

I decided that I would eat only when I was hungry, not when I felt empty.

CHAPTER 41

Checking Out

ZANZIBAR, SEA LEVEL— A FEW DAYS AFTER THE CLIMB

THE AIR OF ZANZIBAR SMELLED of the shell-dotted beach and the perfume of flowers that surrounded the white walls and blue tiles of the resort. There were ample pillows and chairs for lounging. It was just the kind of relaxing spot we needed.

At the front desk, the host asked me if I was married, twice. Despite my response, he asked for my number or my e-mail address. I just smiled.

I had been to the front desk to book a massage for later that afternoon. I returned to our table where our Tusker beers were glowing in the lunchtime sun. I bragged a little about the flirtatious hotel staff.

"Now you're some hot mama," Tracey said. It felt kind of nice, for once, to be admired by them. I felt worthy of their attention. I probably lost ten pounds from the week of exertion. I had to tighten my belt a few notches. It wasn't much, but I wanted to keep going. I smirked a little and settled back into the woven chair. I shifted back and forth in the roominess of it. I slurped down a beer and headed to the massage room.

As I lay on the table, I felt comfortable under the sheet. My legs felt strong. I carried the air of a warrior. The ocean breeze billowed into the open-air room. Still, I was afraid someone would see me through the curtain that danced to and fro.

The massage therapist came in and smiled softly. Then she lifted the sheet to work on my legs. This contact with my body felt nurturing.

"Wow. You are beautiful," the woman said. "If you lived here, your husband would have to guard you with a gun."

"Aw, come on," I said, blushing, my voice muffled by the table.

"No, really. You are lucky to be who you are," she said. She dug her hands into my legs, through the fat, to massage the muscle below.

"These legs are strong," she said. "They have carried you all this way. They will take you far."

CHAPTER 42

Coming Home

SUMMIT, NJ, 374 FEET

THE RAIN POUNDED ON THE windshield and my head spun.

I had just spent fourteen hours in a plane—from Kilimanjaro Airport to Amsterdam and then to JFK. The two-hour cab ride from JFK to my home in Summit, New Jersey, was the final stretch. I hauled my own duffle bag to the side door and let myself in. I could barely drag it down the five stairs to the laundry room. It thumped like a dead body all the way down. My laundry, as steamy and stinky as it was, could wait. The worst of it was concealed within the Ziploc bags my daughter had decorated for me. I thought she would like to see that her stick figures had made a safe return, even if we'd toss them the instant after she saw them since they had become biohazardous. My husband and daughter were due to arrive home from Indiana an hour later.

I lay in bed—feeling a sense of vertigo—dizzy from being still. I closed my eyes and enjoyed the four walls around me. The ceiling above me. The smells of home: ginger hand lotion near my bed, my husband's scent on our sheets. My daughter's shoes strewn across the room.

But I was too excited to rest for long, so I got up to see if there was something to eat. I wasn't really hungry. It was a reflex, opening the cabinet and scanning the contents. But since I wasn't hungry, I closed the cabinet. Just that simple movement felt powerful and strong. It was a step, a small one, to taking better care of myself.

Then the doorbell rang. I could see my daughter's straight bangs as she jumped up and down, trying to see me through the front window. She loved ringing the doorbell as we searched for our keys.

I ran to the door and hugged my family. I felt their love through every layer of my being. I saw my husband and welled up as we held each other, my daughter tugging on my leg.

I was home.

Last Gorge

WATER POUNDED DOWN THREE HUNDRED feet to the lower gorge of Bushkill Falls. It surged beneath the bridge like a thousand fire hoses on full blast.

My husband and now-four-year-old daughter walked ahead of me and leaned on the wooden railing to watch the water rumbling like a rocket tail.

"Careful. Not so close to the edge," I said, mothering from behind. I tried to keep my voice above the noise of the water while not disturbing anyone else's nature experience (even though I had seen a few people on their cell phones).

We had met friends at Bushkill Falls, the "Niagara Falls of Pennsylvania," for a picnic and a hike. We started with homemade Tibetan food made by my friend, a former chef, who had joined us with his wife and two teenage children. I felt satiated and happy before a two-mile walk around the park.

I balanced between one hiking pole and the railing. I had just started to notice my center of gravity was off—that's what happens when you're six months pregnant.

The perpetual flow of water kept the terrain, mostly wooden walkways, moist and mossy, so I was careful. The mist from the water drifted on my face and I smiled with gratitude. I was glad that I'd come. Despite my condition, still overweight and pregnant, I wanted to make sure I kept hiking and exercising. This time, I hadn't gained any extra weight as I carried another healthy girl in my belly. I felt pretty great. So much so, I often forgot I was pregnant.

To be wholly surrounded by the awe-inspiring sights of Bushkill Falls—the trees balancing on the mountainsides, the bridges suspended above the roaring waters, moss in chartreuse tufts—I felt peace and happiness. In a gorge, there is nowhere to go but up.

MY PATH SINCE MY FINAL trek up Mount Kilimanjaro hasn't been perfect. But I feel like I'm in a better place. There are fewer binges. There is more beauty. More deciding which parts of my past to carry with me.

I wish I could say I lost another one hundred pounds. But the mountain didn't cure me, though it helped me understand where I've been. That's the first step in realizing where I need to go.

My father, my molester, my childhood burn, and every lousy experience in my past have made me who I am. But I need to put the bad stuff aside to live the life I desire, a life filled with travel, adventure, and love. It's a lot easier to walk, no matter where I am on the scale, without carrying around all that junk. No bag of candy, no pint (or half gallon) of ice cream, will change the fact that it's easier to walk without the baggage.

"We're on an adventure!" Anna exclaimed, heading to the stairs to the next set of falls, bouncing up and down in pure joy.

"We sure are," I replied, and followed her lead, ready for whatever came next.

I was full.

Acknowledgments

WRITING A BOOK IS A lot like a trek up Kilimanjaro. It is an arduous journey that takes a lot of support along the way.

Without my family, this project wouldn't have been possible. From cheerleaders to book readers—you have helped me be the best I can be.

Thank you to Global Alliance for Africa (globalallianceafrica.org) for providing this experience, and to the brave souls—Stacey, Sally, and Tracey—for being willing to take this journey with me. Thank you to all of our sponsors, who helped us move mountains to support AIDS orphans.

I have immense gratitude for Sydney Clover and Sharon Dennis of Reel World Productions, who hiked up the mountain to document it. Thank you to Scott Farquharson, Derek Wan, Jessica Devra Ferstand, and the late Denise Cramsey for guidance along the way.

Our guides Kenedy and Michael and a crew of nearly forty porters made this trip possible. Thank you for carrying what we could not.

Writers need colleagues who can push them to the next level. There have been so many teachers, mentors, and classmates who have inspired me along the way. Specifically, for this book, Paula Derrow served as my mentor and muse in her amazing Connecticut glass-bottom gazebo retreat. wFrom there, my writing group, Addie Morfoot, Dionne Ford, and Pari Chang, kept me on track. Thank you to my literary match-maker, Sue Shapiro.

Thank you to my brave and fearless Chamonix tribe, Angi Sullins, Roz Bellamy, Tamara Burrows, Heather Eves, Kelly Green, Meghan Smith, Ashley Petry, Suzanne Lerner, Elizabeth Koster, Melina Ragazas, Kate Marck, and Jacey Choy, as well as Butler University's Mike Dahlie, for making my final push of the project so special.

I have so much gratitude for dear Cheryl Strayed, who has pushed me to be brave and to write for years. Thank you for being so generous with knowledge, advice, and love as I finished my manuscript. I have never known someone with so much heart for the craft of writing and those who practice it.

Countless people believed in me on my fitness journey—Heather, Monica, Diane, and Reina to name a few. Thank you for helping me stay on the right path.

There have been many champions for this story, such as my agent Kim Perel and the whole team at Seal Press, especially Krista Lyons. Thank you for embracing *Gorge* and helping me shine.

Dear friends, including Tessa, Suzanne, Megan, Julia, and Jessica, as well as my stellar colleagues at Monaco Lange, helped me through the emotional swells of this dream with laughter and love.

To follow Kara's adventures or even join her along the way,
visit www.kararichardsonwhitely.com

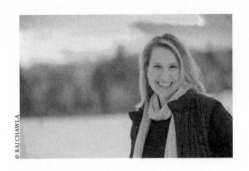

© RAJ CHAWLA

About the Author

KARA RICHARDSON WHITELY MOVES MOUNTAINS. She has hiked Mount Kilimanjaro three times while weighing as much as 300 pounds to raise money for Global Alliance for Africa. Her most recent trek up Africa's highest peak was filmed for a documentary and is the subject of *Gorge*.

Kara, who is also a motivational public speaker, plus-sized fitness advocate, and professional content developer, has written for *Self, Everyday with Rachael Ray,* and *Runner's World* magazines. She was recently featured on *Oprah's Lifeclass,* was an *Outside* magazine 127 Defining Moments finalist, and has been written about in *Redbook* and *American Hiker* magazines. She is also the author of *Fat Woman on the Mountain* and is an American Hiking Society ambassador.

Kara lives in Summit, N.J. with her husband, Chris, and two daughters.

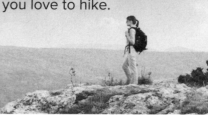

AMERICAN HIKING SOCIETY

Protecting the places you love to hike.

hike.

American Hiking Society gives voice to the more than 50 million Americans who hike and is the only national organization that promotes and protects foot trails, the natural areas that surround them and the hiking experience. Our work is inspiring and challenging, and is built on three pillars:

Policy & Advocacy: We work with Congress and federal agencies to ensure funding for trails, the preservation of natural areas, and the protection of the hiking experience.

Volunteer, Outreach & Education Programs: We organize and coordinate nationally recognized programs, including Volunteer Vacations, Families on Foot and National Trails Day®, which help keep our trails open, safe, and enjoyable.

Trail Grants & Assistance: We support trail clubs and hiking organizations by providing technical assistance, resources, and grant funding so that trails and trail corridors across the country are maintained and preserved.

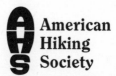

American Hiking Society You too can help and support these efforts! Visit **www.AmericanHiking.org** to become an American Hiking Society member today.

1424 Fenwick Lane, Silver Spring, MD 20910 | 1-800-972-8608
www.AmericanHiking.org | info@americanhiking.org